Giving Evidence at a Mental Health Tribunal

This practical and accessibly written guide introduces what practitioners need to know about Mental Health Tribunals, covering the status of the tribunal, its processes, and the evidence that is required from witnesses. Members of the multidisciplinary team in mental healthcare may have a legal duty to provide oral and written evidence at First-Tier Tribunals (mental health). The tribunal acts as a key safeguard in the provision of mental health care under the Mental Health Act 1983 (as amended 2007) and it is important that all clinicians contributing evidence understand their role and responsibilities. Helping readers to understand what is required of them as witnesses, and to appreciate the extent of the tribunal's powers, this book provides invaluable information about expected best practice and relevant skills, such as distinguishing between an informed opinion and conjecture.

This text is an essential reference for mental health practitioners and students from a range of professions, including nursing, social work, law, occupational therapy, medicine, and psychology.

Toyin Okitikpi is a qualified social worker with over 40 years' experience in the field of social work and social welfare both as a practitioner and as an academic. He currently sits on several tribunals, and he is an external examiner for Tavistock Portman Foundation and University of East London. He has been involved in research and has written and co-authored academic publications that explore practice-related areas.

Herbert Mwebe is a registered mental health nurse and independent prescriber. He has a combined experience of working clinically and in education of over 20 years. He has written and co-authored academic publications in mental health. He is a specialist advisor to the Care Quality Commission and sits on the First-Tier Mental Health Tribunal as a specialist member. He is an external examiner at Bournemouth University.

Helen Rees is a registered nurse and health visitor. She has worked in mental health nursing education since 2012 and currently holds the role of Professional Nurse Educator Lead for Priory group. Helen currently sits on Mental Health Tribunals as a specialist member and is a steering committee member for the Royal College of Nursing.

Giving Evidence at a Mental Health Tribunal

A Professionals' Handbook

Edited by Toyin Okitikpi, Herbert Mwebe, and Helen Rees

Routledge
Taylor & Francis Group

LONDON AND NEW YORK

Designed cover image: The editors

First published 2026
by Routledge
4 Park Square, Milton Park, Abingdon, Oxon OX14 4RN

and by Routledge
605 Third Avenue, New York, NY 10158

Routledge is an imprint of the Taylor & Francis Group, an informa business

© 2026 selection and editorial matter, Edited by Toyin Okitikpi, Herbert Mwebe, and Helen Rees; individual chapters, the contributors

British Library Cataloguing-in-Publication Data
A catalogue record for this book is available from the British Library

ISBN: 9781041064664 (hbk)
ISBN: 9781041064657 (pbk)
ISBN: 9781003635543 (ebk)

DOI: 10.4324/9781003635543

Typeset in Times New Roman
by Newgen Publishing UK

Contents

PART II

Tribunal, Law, and Practice 79

PART III

Evidence in Brief 91

About the Editors

Toyin Okitikpi was a principal lecturer and course director in social work. Having started in residential care he qualified as a generic social worker and worked in the field for many years. His interests include social work education, the importance of education in the lives of children and young people, refugee and asylum-seeking children and their families, social integration, and cohesion, working with children of mixed parentage and interracial/multi-cultural families and their experiences. Currently he sits on several tribunals including the Mental Health Tribunal, the Complementary and Natural Healthcare Council, Employment Tribunal, and the Ministry of Defence Service Complaints Appeals Board. He is a PhD; Professional and Practitioner Doctorate external examiner. He is also a Trustee of Primary Shakespeare Company and Turner Schools Academy Trust.

Herbert Mwebe is an Associate Professor of Mental Health and a Senior Teaching Fellow in the School of Life and Health Sciences. He leads a team of mental health nurse academics in the planning and delivery of pre- and post-reg Mental Health programmes, including CPD. Herbert's teaching and research interests focus on best practice relating to parity of esteem, with reference to improving physical health outcomes in SMI, appropriate, safe, and effective use of psychopharmacological agents, and recovery approaches. He has worked in various higher education and NHS settings, including general practice, secondary, and primary care services. He is a specialist clinical advisor to the CQC, supporting with inspections of community and hospital MH settings. He sits on His Majesty's Courts and Tribunal Service. The First-Tier Mental Health Tribunal as a Specialist Panel Member. He is an editorial board member for the *British of Journal of Mental Health Nursing* and an External Examiner at Bournemouth University on a range of CPD modules. He is a peer reviewer for various journals including *Mental Health Practice* (RCNi). As QAA registrant visitor, Herbert undertakes the delivery of quality assurance services to the Nursing and Midwifery Council (NMC). Herbert is a co-director and lead for Education and Training for a CIC diaspora health association, Uganda Nurses, and Midwives Association UK.

Helen Rees is a registered nurse and health visitor. She has worked in mental health nursing education since 2012 and currently holds the role of Professional Nurse Educator Lead for Priory group. Helen teaches across a range of topics; areas of interest include children and young people's mental health, mental health law, and the reduction of coercion in healthcare. Helen is a steering committee member of the RCN mental health forum and a specialist judiciary member. Helen is a published author in several nursing areas and is a reviewer across several nursing journals. Helen sits on the approval panel for several national grant awards and is part of the accreditation team for the Royal College of Nursing.

Contributors

Joanne Briggs has been a salaried judge of the Mental Health Tribunal since February 2009, having been appointed as a fee-paid mental health Judge in 2002. Jo is a member of the Restricted Patient Panel and is the Liaison Judge for tribunal members living and working in Sussex and Kent. Jo completed a Master of Philosophy degree by research in mental health law and policy, working with MIND's legal department and its archives. She was a barrister for sixteen years, mainly practising in public law family and crime. She also represented local authorities and patients in complex mental health cases.

Jo has an MA in creative writing. A memoir about her early life is due to be published in 2025.

Andy Cook is a consultant clinical psychologist working within forensic healthcare. She works with people with severe and enduring mental health problems who have posed a significant risk to others and/or self, and who often have complex trauma histories. She undertakes assessments of risk and mental health and delivers treatment and therapy. She has specialised in systemic and group interventions, including family intervention, restorative practice, psychodynamic reflective groups, staff reflective practice and critical incident support. She is interested in the repair of relational bonds and the crucial role of relationships in working towards recovery and resilience.

Barbara Deacon-Hedges passion for improving mental health started when she was a young child. She began her social work career in London working in emergency intake children's homes working with children in trauma from physical and mental abuse. She has since worked in adult social care and health services in England for over 40 years mainly with those who made use of mental health services. Prior to community care being rolled out, she was asked to develop a pilot programme of education training and work opportunities for mental health service users. This ended up as a service model that was used and is still used in the UK and aboard. Barbara moved on to national inspection and practice improvement both in the UK and other countries. Barbara has been a non-executive director of several mental health charities. Outside of work she is busy learning how to garden having been recently told that the "honeysuckle" she planted in several places was actually bindweed. Undeterred, her belief is to garden and to believe in tomorrow.

Russell Foster is a London-based Consultant Psychiatrist and worked in academic gastroenterology before completing his psychiatric training at the Maudsley Hospital in London. He holds dual accreditation in General Adult Psychiatry as well as Liaison Psychiatry. He holds qualifications from universities in Canada, Norway, Hong Kong, England, Wales, and Scotland. His credentials include a PhD in biochemistry, and master's degrees in toxicology, the philosophy of mental health and public administration as well as an LLM in mental health law. He has around 100 publications including a 500-page book about blood tests in psychiatry.

Kristian Garsed was called to the Bar (England & Wales), by Inner Temple (2006) and practised at 4KBW from 2006 – 2011. In 2011 Kristian joined the Regulatory Legal Team at the Nursing and Midwifery Council (NMC), initially as a lawyer, and then a senior lawyer. In 2014 he was called to the Bar of Northern Ireland. Kristian has been a Regulation Adviser (RA) in Professional Practice at the NMC since 2016. He is currently the RA for North-East England & Yorkshire and the Humber. He is a former fee-paid Employment Judge (London East Employment Tribunal), 2021 – 2023 and has been sitting as a fee-paid First-Tier Tribunal Judge (Health, Education, and Social Care Chamber) in the Mental Health jurisdiction since 2021.

Philip Jones is a senior lecturer in public health at Nottingham Trent University. A qualified mental health nurse, his speciality was assertive outreach work with focus on the engagement and the management of some of the more difficult to engage and risky clientele living within the community. Teaching since 2012, he was course leader at Birmingham City University and a member of the course leadership team that launched the future nurse curriculum, where he had specific responsibility for around 500 mental health students. Prior to BCU he was at Middlesex University on the Mental health BSc programme and played a significant role in developing and implementing what was then the new curriculum. He has completed level 7 qualifications in development management, an MBA and an MSc in systems think in practice, amongst others. He contributed to a variety of education projects in the developing world and to work combating human trafficking in Southeast Asia. He remains committed to social justice within the UK but also more widely with a growing global perspective. He is a charted fellow of the Chartered Management Institute and a chartered fellow of the Institute for Leadership.

Shazad Malik qualified as a solicitor in 2004 and as a Higher Courts Advocate (All Proceedings) in 2010. He has worked as an immigration advocate, representing before the [then] Immigration Appellate Authority. He has experience in various areas of law, including crime, prison law, community care, judicial review, and European Court of Human Rights. He was awarded Law Society Mental Health Panel Accreditation in 2005. He founded Appleton's Solicitors in partnership, in 2018. He continues to advise and represent in relation to the Mental Health Act 1983 (as amended) and the Mental Capacity Act 2005. He sits as a Police Misconduct and Police Appeals Tribunal (PAT) member and has previously been a member of the Independent Police Ethics Committee Member. He is a fee-paid (part-time) Judge of the First-Tier Tribunal in the Health, Education, and Social Care Chamber (HESC) and regularly sits in the Mental Health Jurisdiction.

Ruairi Mulhern is a senior lecturer at Middlesex University. Trained as an RMN at Purdysburn Hospital, Belfast, in 1990 before moving to London in the mid 1990's. Further study and career were based in Camden & Islington as a Community Mental Health Nurse, BiA and AMHP. Transferred over to nurse education in 2015.

Jennifer Oates is a mental health nurse academic with a clinical background in liaison mental health and community mental health. Jenny has expertise in healthcare regulation and mental health law, through previous appointments with the Nursing and Midwifery Council, The General Medical Council, and the Care Quality Commission. She holds a master's in Social Research from the University of Leeds and a master's in law from the University of Manchester. Her PhD was on the mental health and subjective wellbeing in UK mental health nurses. She continues to research and practice in the field of the mental wellbeing in healthcare professionals and students. Her current role is Lead for Wellbeing in the School of Health Sciences at the University of Surrey. Jenny is a Specialist Member of First-Tier Tribunals – Mental Health.

Ahmad F Ramjhun, BSc (Hons), PGCE, Dip Sp ED, MSc, MBA, MA (Ed), EdD, AFBPsS, CPsychol, Reg Psychol. Consultant Psychologist and Specialist Tribunal Member (Mental Health, SENDIST and DDC), Health Education and Social Care Chamber and Social Entitlement Chamber.

Gareth Rees works as a consultant psychiatrist, medical appraiser, and college tutor in the mental health division of Birmingham Women's and Children's NHS Foundation Trust. He has been a member of the Royal College of Psychiatrists since 2012 and was awarded a Master of Laws (Healthcare Ethics and Law) from the University of Manchester in 2016. Dr Rees also completed a Postgraduate Certificate in Medical Education with the University of Dundee in 2018 and became an Honorary Clinical Lecturer (University of Birmingham) in 2021. He has published journal articles and book chapters on the themes of medical education and the Mental Health Act 1983 (amended 2007) and has been a Medical Member of the First-Tier Tribunal (Mental Health) since 2021.

Jane Roberts is a consultant forensic psychologist currently working in a secure forensic hospital. She is registered with the Health and Care Professions Council (HCPC) as a forensic psychologist in the UK. She has 20 years of experience of working in prisons, forensic mental health hospitals, and with service users in the community. She has worked with people with offending histories, including people with mental illness, experience of trauma, and people who may be considered to meet a diagnosis of personality disorder. Jane also provides independent expert witness assessments.

Amy Rushen qualified as a solicitor in 2004 and specialised in family law following qualification. She then moved into teaching, with a focus on vocational legal education. She went on to lead undergraduate and postgraduate programmes at a number of universities including The University of Law, Kaplan Law School, and BPP University Law School, as well as being appointed a Senior Fellow of the Higher Education Academy. She now sits as a Fee Paid Judge of the First-Tier Tribunal in both the Mental Health Tribunal and the Special Educational Needs and Disability Tribunal, as well as sitting as a Deputy District Judge.

Catherine Stobbs is a registered adult nurse working in the Central Priory Nurse Education team. Cath has a clinical background of accident and emergency nursing and leading physical health support in Mental Health Services within Priory Healthcare. Cath recently gained a PGCE from Bolton University where she lectured and tutored RMN Apprentices to complete their Nursing Degree, gaining a fellowship to Advanced Higher Education. Cath's current role is Priory Nurse Lecturer.

Lorraine Summers is an expert with over 30 years' experience in the MH system. Previously a volunteer at Whittington Hospital, she currently is an advocate and a visiting lecturer at Middlesex University.

Victoria Tracey is a mental health nurse academic with a clinical background in inpatient acute, PICU, and forensic settings and community mental health. Victoria is an independent nurse prescriber and is a fellow of the University of Greater Manchester.
Victoria' current role is a nurse lecturer at the University of Greater Manchester and a nurse educator within The Priory.

John S Watts is a child and adolescent psychiatrist working in the NHS, and also a medical member of the Mental Health Tribunal Service. He has an interest in the interface between the law and clinical practice, and in consent, capacity, and competence in the under 18s. He has co-authored academic articles in clinical and legal journals. He has worked in clinical practice for nearly 30 years, with a brief stint in medicines research.

Preface

This book was born out of the desire to enable and support mental health professionals to provide the necessary information required at the Mental Health Tribunal hearing. It is worth acknowledging that giving evidence at such a formal and imposing environment is not necessarily comfortable or easy for witnesses. It is generally taken for granted that the tribunal should try, as best as possible, to create a welcoming and non-threatening atmosphere to encourage and facilitate the full participation of all those in attendance, in particular the patients and their relatives. It is assumed that the members of the treating team giving evidence at the tribunal are experienced professionals and are therefore well versed in such formal settings. There is often very little consideration extended to them as they are deemed to be the detaining authority who need to prove their case. The contention advanced in this volume is that, for all concerned, including the professionals, giving evidence in front of a tribunal panel can be a nerve-racking experience, even for the most seasoned practitioner. At some level it is a professionally exposing environment because it places the practices and treatment of people, whose case is being heard, under scrutiny. It requires professionals to provide cogent explanation, with evidence, of their treatment plan and why someone should remain detained under section rather than as a voluntary patient. It expects the treating team to speak with direct knowledge and understanding of the patients' current mental state, their diagnosis, and prognosis. It may seem an otiose or obvious point to make but it is nevertheless worth stating from the outset that tribunals are specialist judicial bodies with legal powers, as set out under the Tribunals, Courts, and Enforcement Act 2007. There is often a confusion, even amongst some representatives, as to whether the mental health tribunal's approach is adversarial, like some other tribunals such as Employment and Land registry, or inquisitorial. The uncertainty of the tribunal's approach is to some extent understandable since it is taken for granted that the patient and their representative would be challenging and trying to undermine the treating team's case for detention. While the patient and their representatives may indeed view the system as adversarial, for the mental health tribunal panel, the approach is more inquisitorial, as they aim to get to the heart of the matter through an extensive examination and investigation of all the evidence available to them, including questioning members of the treating team, the patient and other witnesses. In effect, the tribunal is a self-contained judicial entity with the powers to make decisions and give directions. The function of the tribunal is put succinctly and simply by Mind organisation in its general advice to people seeking information about what to expect from a tribunal, (mind.org.uk, 2023). It proffered to patients enquiring that the tribunal would:

- Look at their mental health and how well they are doing
- Speak to them and the professional involved in their care, and
- Ask for up-to-date reports.

They would use the information to decide if they:

- Still fit the conditions for being sectioned, or
- Should be discharged from their section and possibly leave hospital, (mind.org.uk// mentalhealthtribunal13/11/23).

In essence, the tribunal hears applications and references for people who are detained under the Mental Health Act 1983 (as amended by the Mental Health Act 2007) or are living in the community following the making of a guardianship order, conditional discharge, or a community treatment order.

The central theme of this book is to support mental health professionals and treating teams and to instil a degree of confidence about their role and what is required of them at the tribunal hearing. Too often practitioners seem unsure of both the status of the tribunal and the kind of evidence that is required from them. In some cases, there is uncertainty as to whether the hearing should be viewed as a conference, a review meeting, managers review, or an extension of the multidisciplinary team meeting. It is not unusual for some professionals giving evidence to attend the tribunal unprepared. In some cases, at best, they have very little knowledge of the patient's history, circumstance, current mental state, or the environment into which they may be discharged. At worst, they have shown no professional curiosity about the patient or their situation and are unable to provide even the most basic information about the patient's mental state and circumstance. Despite having access to previous and recent reports, medical notes, medicine charts, ward round and MDT meetings and opportunities to contact the patient, either remotely or face-to-face to assess and find out about their situation prior to the tribunal hearing, or ascertained the views of the nearest relative, often no such general inquiries are undertaken. It is worth acknowledging, in fairness to some of the professionals that they are sometimes required to attend hearings at short notice, because of staff shortages, changes of shift patterns, planned leaves, and unexpected absences or patients have been moved to their unit due to lack of bed spaces in the patient's home area. There are examples of professional witnesses only discovering that they were attending and giving evidence perhaps a day or a couple of hours before the start of the hearing. The short attendance notice, it could be argued, is unhelpful as it affords the professional concerned insufficient time and opportunity to get to peruse the available reports in detail and get to know the patient and at the same time acquire the level of knowledge and understanding that would enable them to give evidence, with any degree of confidence, at the tribunal. They are required to represent their professional opinion and recommendations based on their knowledge, assessment, treatment, care and observation of the patient yet they may feel disempowered and professionally embarrassed because, as they do not know the patient well enough, they are ill-prepared and unable to answer the questions put to them by the tribunal panel and the patient's representative.

The aim of this book is to encourage practitioners to see the hearing as a formal process in an informal setting where they are required to give written and oral evidence as a member of the treating team. They are expected to know and understand the qualitative difference between the various terminologies, for example: necessity, desirable, nature, degree, insight, appropriate treatment, power of recall, conditions, who is the nearest relative, capacity, consent to treatment, seeking information from the nearest relative without the patient's consent, the three limbs of risk assessment.

The book is in three parts and, although each section is self-contained, the chapters can be read out of sequence. As those involved in the mental health service would be already aware there are a number of policies and guidance in place to support staff working in the field. For example, there are report guidelines that set out clearly what is required in a report for the Mental Health Tribunal. Practitioners are expected to follow the practice guidelines and make use of the appropriate templates which are freely available. This volume does deviate from the policies and guidelines already in place but instead it attempts to encourage practitioners to develop a better understanding of their role and responsibility at the tribunal and to be mindful of the purpose and focus of the tribunal. Those involved in the case and giving evidence should attend fully prepared to answer searching and, potentially challenging, questions about the patient's mental state, the range of treatment they are receiving, the risk they may pose and the range of provision and support available in the community, should the tribunal be minded to discharging the section or support a conditional discharge.

Part one is about practitioners' role and the articulation and presentation of the range of treatments available to people in their care. Although the section will explore and discuss symptoms, medication and other forms of interventions, the chapters focus on the importance of practitioners' knowledge and understanding of the day-to-day treatment regime and their long-term plans for the patient. At the tribunal hearing, mental health professionals are expected to demonstrate a good understanding of the symptomology (degree, chronicity, symptom variations) relating to the course and nature of mental disorders. It is this knowledge and application that they will need to rely on to engage and be able to respond to questions raised by the tribunal panel and the patient's representative.

Chapter 1 provides a general overview of mental disorder and the symptomology that gives rise to the different categorisations. There is a brief, but helpful, discussion on the difference between nature and degree, the three limbs of the risk assessment and how insight should be assessed. Following the exploration of mental disorder, the focus of the next five chapters shifts onto the range of treatments that are available and can be accessed by patients.

In Chapter 2 there is a general discussion and an overview of the different types of medication administered for mental disorder. Although the chapter does not provide a description of every medication that is available, it does highlight the different class of medicines, their efficacy and possible side effects.

In Chapter 3 the discussion is about the therapeutic provisions available for both in hospital and community-based patients. It attempts to explore the range of therapeutic services on offer as well as reference to how these are accessed.

Chapter 4 focuses on the range of activities that are needed to support daily living and encourages health and wellbeing. It explains why occupational therapy is important and how it could help to improve social relationships, enhance people's quality of life as well equip people with the necessary skills and knowledge to cope with day-to-day living.

Chapter 5 discusses the nursing care that patients generally have access to in hospital and in the community, in some cases. It highlights the range of support and care available as well as the medicine regime and compliance considerations. It explores practical support in place to assess, monitor, evaluate and treat patients both in hospital and in the community.

Chapter 6 explores community provisions that are available, including home-treatment teams, crisis team and the extent of mental health services involvement with the patient. It considers the general support and social network in the patient's locality.

Chapter 7 explores the process by which people are compulsorily admitted into hospital following an assessment. It looks at both restricted and non-restricted cases and the criteria that informs such detentions. The chapter effectively considers the legal framework and other considerations for compulsory admission.

The aims of **Part two**, Chapter 8, is to set out, in broad terms, the purpose and function of the mental health tribunal. It highlights the legislative framework within which the tribunal operates and discusses the application of its guiding principles. It explores the criteria that informs the panel's approach and the nature of the decision they ae required to make.

The focus of **Part three** is about the evidence that are expected to be provided by witnesses at a Mental Health Tribunal hearing.

Chapter 9 is an overview of what is involved and required of all the witnesses when giving evidence at the tribunal. It discusses the etiquette, requirements and quality of the evidence that is expected.

Chapter 10 discusses the key points that are required from the nurse's evidence and why it is important to provide the collective view of the care team. It highlights the need to be able to provide specific examples of symptoms that are documented in reports and talk about the day-to-day functioning of the patient, their medication regime and compliance, section 17 leave arrangement, incidents, insight, progress, relationships with others, and their response to treatment.

In Chapter 11, sets out who can give evidence, and the nature of the information required. Although the evidence of all witnesses carries equal weight, particular attention is paid to the responsible clinician's evidence as their judgement and opinion gives the panel a general overview of the patient's diagnosis, current mental state, risks, prognosis and how they are responding to treatment.

In Chapter 12 the consideration is about the role and expectations of the care coordinator and the community team in supporting the patient. The chapter highlights the key points that care coordinators should present to the tribunal as their evidence could play a decisive role in the panel's decision on whether to discharge, using their discretionary powers, even though the patient might have met the criteria for continued detention. For example, there should be information presented about the social care plan, the support regime in the community, discharge plan and any proposed aftercare provisions.

In Chapter 13, The chapter attempts to explores the importance of the patient's evidence and also the role and responsibilities of the nearest relative and the patient's advocate at the hearing. Often there are uncertainties about the position of the advocate and the nearest relative and what is required of them, if anything, at the tribunal hearing.

Chapter 14 looks at the role of the patient's representative and what it is that they are seeking to get out of the tribunal hearing. Although, in most instances, they are working under instruction from the patient (their client), there are also occasions when they have to act in the best interest of the patient as they have sought to be appointed by the tribunal because their client lacks capacity.

Acknowledgements

We are grateful to Grace McInnes and Madaline Cherry-Moreton at Routledge/Taylor & Francis for their help and support. We would like to say a special thanks to all the contributors who despite their busy schedules were very generous with their time in committing their thoughts and ideas to paper, we owe then a debt of gratitude. Also, a mention to Matthew Mwebe for rising to the challenge of designing the front cover. Finally, we greatly appreciated the encouragement of Julia Morris and the team at Critical Publishing for accepting our initial idea of a volume to support those giving evidence at a Mental Health Tribunal.

Part I

Introduction, Mental Disorder, and Treatment

1 Understanding Mental Disorder

Russell Foster

Introduction – What is Mental Disorder?

It should be noted that there is a substantial literature in this field and an ongoing debate that remains regarding what constitutes mental disorder, with, for example, Varga (2015), p. 10) suggesting that:

> psychiatry has a unique position 'torn between' (medical) science and the humanities, and therefore faces unique methodological challenges with regard to both clinical practice and research
>
> (Varga, 2015, p.10)

With this given context, the current chapter aims to consider this concept practically and pragmatically, concentrating on clinical and legal concepts relevant to the Mental Health Tribunal. Although superficially straight-forward, this question is highly complex, for example, as noted by Bolton in his 310-page book, where he attempted to provide a definitive answer – but ultimately could not:

> there [is] no stable reality or concept of mental disorder, it breaks up into many, quite different kinds, some reminiscent of an old idea or mental illness, others nothing like this at all. This instability and fragmentation corresponds to diversity in the phenomena, in current clinical services and in current terminology. I would have settled for one clear proposal as to what mental disorder really is but couldn't find one.
>
> (Bolton, 2008, p. viii)

Case law accepts there is no single definition of mental disorder (for example, R. (on the application of B) v Ashworth Hospital Authority [2005] UKHL 20; [2005] 2 All E.R., para 31 and Winterwerp v Netherlands (1979) E.H.R.R. 387, para 37) and suggests that it is essentially clinical judgement as to what constitutes mental disorder (Attia v British Gas [1998] Q.B. 304).

Another difficulty in defining mental disorder comes from varying viewpoints: is mental disorder a philosophical, social, political, clinical, or legal entity? Controversially, a number of authors suggest that there is actually no such thing as mental disorder, with a seminal work, "The Myth of Mental Illness", (Szasz, 1961), proposing that mental disorder is a social construct with no biological basis. Breaking down the term mental disorder into its constituent parts and considering each of these separately also suggests that the concept of "mental" (that is, to do with the "mind") is problematic, due to the lack of any definitive definition of what the mind is, (Schaafsma *et al.*, 2015), or what constitutes a "disorder" (Tait, 2010). Mental disorder

DOI: 10.4324/9781003635543-2

remains a complex concept philosophically, but helpfully there are legal and clinical definitions which provide some clarity. So again, what is mental disorder? The following points offer some helpful guidance, starting with the legal definition of the concept:

1. According to the MHA 2003, (amended 2007), section 1(2), mental disorder is defined as, "any disorder or disability of the mind". It is noted here that this definition is problematic, given the lack of any universally accepted definition of "mind" or "disorder" as noted above. This definition is broad, does not require a specific diagnosis, and excludes drug and alcohol dependency (unless also accompanied by or associated with a mental disorder). The presence of a mental disorder will largely be based on clinical evidence, although the law does note that mental disorder is not necessarily present if a person behaves in a manner which may be perceived as irrational, unusual or contrary to prevailing societal views (St George's Healthcare NHS Trust v S [1988] 3 All E.R. 673; R v Deighton [2005] EWCA Crim 3131).

2. The World Health Organization defines mental disorder thus:

> A mental disorder is characterized by a clinically significant disturbance in an individual's cognition, emotional regulation, or behaviour. It is usually associated with distress or impairment in important areas of functioning.
>
> (WHO, 2022, p.1)

Note that this definition excludes aetiology, with physical health disorders not normally deemed mental disorders unless they specifically give rise to disorders of the mind. Hence "brain" disorders, such as epilepsy, would not generally be deemed as mental disorders despite some forms of epilepsy, such as temporal lobe epilepsy, being associated with psychotic symptoms. The interplay of physical and mental health as defined by the MHA is complex and beyond the scope of the current discussion, but has been considered by Wheeler and Ruck Keene (2022). Additionally, distress as commonly understood may be evident in mental disorder but is not necessarily a proxy for mental disorder, (Drapeau *et al.*, 2012), despite its frequent association with mental health presentations.

3. When considering what is *not* a mental disorder, it is useful to consider aetiology, with the Mental Health Code of Practice (2015) definition of "nature" considering "predisposing factors", (see below). Consideration of potential differential diagnoses is an important part of the psychiatric formulation, which is discussed later in this chapter. The related concept of "normality" in relation to mental disorders remains unclear, (Wakefield and First, 2013), and is perhaps less useful than considering a person's baseline functioning through careful history taking and obtaining of collateral evidence.

4. Specific clinical definitions of mental health disorders are presented in diagnostic manuals such as ICD-11 and DSM-5, which classify mental disorders and thereby aim to assist with diagnosis. Reference to a specific diagnosis, be it a "working" diagnosis or one that is confirmed based on a comprehensive history and examination constitutes potentially helpful evidence confirming the presence of a mental disorder, although it is important to understand how this diagnosis is formulated, noting, for example, objective evidence from mental state examination, collateral history and ongoing monitoring and exclusion of non-mental health causes.

Assessing Mental Disorder

Although mental disorders are not the sole preserve of psychiatry, the psychiatric assessment process provides the useful basis for diagnosis and subsequent management and understanding the basis of this.. It is important to note that psychiatry is a medical specialty and that the medical model, which suggests that there is a biological cause for mental disorders, still predominates in clinical practice. Although controversial, this paradigm does imply that considering potential causes and ruling these in or out is an important part of the evaluation.

The assessment process in psychiatry is generally similar to that followed in all medical practice, that is, to obtain a history from the patient, undertake a clinical examination followed by investigations and finally by management, which includes medical and other potential treatments. Medical treatment is defined in the MHA as summarised below. The process aims at identifying symptoms to formulate a clinical impression or working diagnosis which thereby guides management. Taking a psychiatric history involves obtaining information from the patient (as well as collateral information from other sources) as noted in Table 1.1.

There is no single format for history taking and careful questioning will usually elicit the required information, although obtaining all of the required details may not be possible in a single attempt. It is also noted that such interviews may not be fully reliable, (Matarazzo, 1978), nor consistent, and so collateral evidence will need careful consideration.

While in "physical medicine" it is possible to undertake a clinical examination and undertake investigations to obtain objective evidence, evaluation of mental disorders is more complex as there are no clinical signs, (objective features that can be observed by the assessor), specific to any mental disorder. Hence the process requires evaluation of the individual in order to both elicit symptoms of mental disorder, ruling out other causes not associated with mental disorder, and thereby determine a management plan. The key assessment framework is that of the Mental State Examination as summarised in Table 1.2.

Table 1.1 Elements of a Psychiatric History

Domain	Examples of relevant Information
Demographics	Name, age, date of birth, names of any informants and relationship to patient
History of Presenting Complaint	Why patient has presented, what they feel the problem is, the nature of the problem, current severity, other problems, onset, course, and impact;
Past Psychiatric History	Previous diagnoses, admissions, treatment, outcomes;
Past Medical History	Including current/past problems, treatment and impact, smoking, substance use; menstrual/obstetric history for females;
Medication Treatment	Current medication details (names, doses, frequency, how long the patient has been taking these, what last taken, any problems with concordance, how helpful they have been, attitude to continuing, any other treatment, allergies/intolerances;
Social History	Accommodation, who does the patient live with, marital status, relationships, children, work, income, social stressors;
Family History	Details re history of mental disorder in parents, relationship with patient, work, personality, ages/cause of death, siblings, extended family;
Personal History	Mother's pregnancy, birth, early development, problems in childhood such as (separations, emotional problems, and medical problems), education (attendance, behaviour, attainment), work, sexual relationships, marriage, children;
Pre-morbid personality	Character, prevailing mood, interests/hobbies, leisure activities, attitudes, standards, religion;
Forensic history	Criminal record, incarceration, history of trouble with police;

Table 1.2 Summary of the Features of the Mental State Examination

Domain	Examples of Relevant Details
Appearance and Behaviour	General appearance, behaviour, facial expression, self-care, clothing, eye contact, rapport, posture, movements, abnormal movements, gait, mannerisms, habitus, medical signs;
Speech	Rate, quantity, tone, volume, prosody, pitch, stuttering/stammering, perseveration;
Mood	Subjective, objective, affect
'Biological symptoms of Depression'	Sleep, Appetite/weight gain or loss, attention, concentration, anhedonia, diurnal mood variation, self-esteem, libido;
Thought form	Thought disorder, flight of ideas, circumstantial speech, tangentiality, derailing;
Thought content	Perceptual abnormalities, preoccupations, delusions, overvalued ideas, first rank symptoms, obsessive-compulsive phenomena, paranoid/persecutory ideation, anxiety symptoms, derealisation, depersonalisation;
Cognition	Level of consciousness, memory (short- and long-term), orientation (time, place, person), attention, concentration. intelligence, confusion;
Suicidal/self-harm	Current/past history, thoughts, plans, view on whether life is worth living, plans for future, social support;
Insight	Awareness of symptoms, view on whether they feel unwell and why, what they feel the problem is, their view on need for treatment, their view on engagement;

Statutory Criteria – Nature and Degree

Within the MHA there are specific criteria for detention, all of which will need to be met for an individual to be detained under the Act, depending on the section under consideration. The presence of mental disorder is the first fundamental criterion, followed by determining whether nature and/or degree are present. A seminal case defines **Nature** as:

> …the particular mental disorder from which the patient suffers, its chronicity, its prognosis, and the patient's previous response to receiving treatment for the disorder.
>
> (R v Mental Health Review Tribunal for the South Thames Region
> Ex p. Smith [1999] C.O.D. 148)

Chronicity refers to length of time the patient has had the condition and its course (for example, relapsing and remitting). These details can be determined via the history. It should be noted that in a first presentation, with no previous history, it is difficult to argue nature (such as, for example, in the first admission of an individual under section 2). This can include a consideration of whether a patient is likely to relapse quickly if discharged (see, for example, R (Smith) v MHRT South Thames Region (1998) EWHC Admin 832 and Smirek v Williams [2002] M.H.L.R. 38).

Degree is also defined in R v Mental Health Review Tribunal for the South Thames Region Ex p. Smith [1999] C.O.D. 148 as, "the current manifestations of the patient's disorder", (ibid), that is, the current presentation in terms of symptoms. It is useful to consider how these symptoms compare to those on admission as these may change, not least in response to medical treatment. While not included in the definitions of nature and degree, the notion of insight is sometimes included as a measure of both nature and degree, although this remains controversial with no clear consensus on what insight means and how it is assessed, (Guidry-Grimes, 2019).

Statutory Criteria – Risk and Risk Assessment

It is noteworthy that the MHA does not formally define what constitutes risk, and that risk and its assessment are complex and controversial (Fanning 2016). For the current purposes, the

Table 1.3 Summary of Some of the Risks to Health, Safety and Others

Domain	Risk	Notes
Health	Medication non-compliance	Case law confirms that someone on medication for a disorder continues to suffer from that disorder (Devon CC v Hawkins [1967] 2 Q.B. 26 despite lack of symptoms and can still meet the requirement for degree – history of previous relapse will be pertinent here. Note further that in *Smirek v Williams* [*2000*] EWCA Civ 3025 liability to be detained in hospital can be appropriate if evidence shows that the patient would not take medication needed to prevent deterioration unless detained in hospital. This case referred to an individual with a chronic mental disorder.
	Non-engagement	This may be due to factors outwith mental disorder (Dixon *et al.*, 2016), which again will be guided by history
	Self-neglect	May include failure to care for personal hygiene, surroundings, and nutritional intake.
	Substance abuse	Note that both intoxication and withdrawal are relevant here, and that substance abuse can prolong and worse mental disorder and can be associated with risk to safety and protection of others.
	Inability to manage physical health condition due to mental health disorder	
Safety	Self-harm	These may be identified in the clinical interview, in ongoing observations and via collateral history.
	Suicide	
	Vulnerability to exploitation	
	Vulnerability to abuse from others (physical, emotional, violence)	
	Vulnerability to retaliation	
	Absconding	
	Road Safety	
	Risk of radicalisation	
	Risks associated with housing and social circumstances	These may relate to temporary and/or poor-quality housing and social concerns which may increase the risk of neglect
Protection of Others	Assault/physical harm to others	This may include verbal, physical, and emotional abuse and harassment, invective and intentional neglect or provocation of others.
	Risks due to behaviour related to mental disorder	

definition of risk will be that of the usual meaning of the word, that is, the likeliness of an event occurring, noting that these risks relating to a mental health disorder are interpreted as acute risks, that is, risks that are both likely and imminent, as opposed to risks that may likely arise in the longer-term. There is an associated concept of dangerousness, which has been discussed at length in the mental health and criminal law literature (see, for example, de Vries and Bijlsma 2022; Large *et al.*, 2008). While dangerousness remains controversial, it should be noted that danger and risk are not necessarily synonymous, and the former can be interpreted as an extreme form of risk, with risks including a wider-ranging concept.

The MHA Code of practice refers to various risks including suicide, self-harm, self-neglect, deterioration, accidental, reckless, or unintentional jeopardy, and a wide range of other risks may be identified based on individual circumstances. Table 1.3 provides a summary of some of the key risks to health, safety, and protection of others.

Risks to health include both physical and health risks, with a potentially complex interplay between these, as physical health problems may be symptoms or causes of mental disorders and may not be apparent at time of assessment. That said, the MHA can under certain circumstances be used to treat physical disorders connected to mental health conditions as noted in sections 63 and 145 of the MHA. This is also confirmed in case law: B v Croydon Health Authority [1995] 1 All E.R. 683): "ancillary treatment" aimed at relieving symptoms of mental disorder is permissible to avoid the patient causing harm to themselves or alleviating the consequences of the mental disorder.

Risks to mental health are often described as deterioration, non-engagement, non-concordance with treatment, and will be based on history, observation, and ideally collateral evidence, give the complexities of determining and assessing risk, especially for individuals with a first presentation of mental disorder. Risks to safety are related to risk of being harmed if not detained, with a range of these noted in Table 1.3.

As regards protection of others, it should be noted that through contributions from case law, risk need not necessarily be related to the public at large, and may well be related only to a specific individual/individuals, (R. v North West London Mental Health NHS Trust Ex p. Stewart (1996) 39 B.M.L.R. 105).

Assessment of Risk

Although formal risk assessment tools exist, (Department of Health, 2009), none of these is entirely accurate, (Wand, 2011), and anecdotally seldom appear to be used in routine clinical practice. While risk assessment is complex and can be subjective, there is a large amount of published guidance, for example that published by the UK Department of Health (2009), the Royal College of Psychiatrists (2016). Table 1.4 summarises this latter guidance, which may provide useful hints for understanding risk, noting that findings of facts regarding risk will be based on elicited evidence and will be discussed in later chapters of this book.

Insight

In general terms, insight refers to an individual's understanding of their situation, with the "ideal" insightful patient understanding that they have a mental disorder that needs treating, are willing to accept and engage in ongoing treatment, and generally follow the advice of the treating clinician. Insight is problematic as it is not a unitary phenomenon, with, for example, Marková and Berrios (1992), suggesting that the concept is a continuum with a large number of variables. Given its complexity, and the varying interpretation of insight as a potential aspect

Table 1.4 Royal College of Psychiatrists Risk Assessment Factors

Domain	Factor
History	• Previous violence, whether investigated, convicted or unknown to the criminal justice system. • Relationship of violence to mental state. Lack of supportive relationships. • Poor concordance with treatment, discontinuation, or disengagement. Impulsivity. Alcohol or substance use, and the effects of these. • Early exposure to violence or being part of a violent subculture. • Triggers or changes in behaviour or mental state that have occurred prior to previous violence or relapse. • Are risk factors stable or have any changed recently? • Is anything likely to occur that will change the risk? • Evidence of recent stressors, losses, or threat of loss. • Factors that have stopped the person acting violently in the past. • Are the family/carers at risk? • History of domestic violence. • Lack of empathy. • Relationship of violence to personality factors.
Environment	• Risk factors may vary by setting and patient group. • Risk on release from restricted settings. • Consider protective factors or loss of protective factors. • Relational security • Risks of reduced bed capacity and alternatives to admission. • Access to potential victims, particularly individuals identified in mental state abnormalities. • Access to weapons, violent means, or opportunities. • Involvement in radicalisation.
Mental State	• Evidence of symptoms related to threat or control, delusions of persecution by others, or of mind or body being controlled or -interfered with by external forces, or passivity experiences. • Voicing emotions related to violence or exhibiting emotional arousal (e.g. irritability, anger, hostility, suspiciousness, excitement, enjoyment, notable lack of emotion, cruelty, or incongruity). • Specific threats or ideas of retaliation. • Grievance thinking. • Thoughts linking violence and suicide (homicide–suicide). • Thoughts of sexual violence. • Evolving symptoms and unpredictability. Signs of psychopathy. • Restricted insight and capacity. • Patient's own narrative and view of their risks to others. • What does the person think they are capable of? • Do they think they could kill? • Beware 'invisible' risk factors.
Information from Other Sources	• Has everyone with relevant information been consulted? This includes carers, criminal records, Police National Computer markers, and probation reports
Risk Formulation	• How serious is the risk? • How immediate is the risk? • Is the risk specific or general? • How volatile is the risk? • What are the signs of increasing risk? Which specific treatment, and which management plan, can best reduce the risk?

(*Continued*)

Table 1.4 (Continued)

Domain	Factor
Management Plan	• Is the person capacitous? • Will the person engage and how much? • Is it possible to agree a safety plan? (Record lack of engagement.) • Is home treatment feasible or is admission necessary? • What community supports are available (e.g. family, carers, community mental health nurses, approved mental health professionals, probation)? • Do carers and family feel supported and do they have easy, timely access to help? • What psychological interventions might be helpful? • What level of observation is required? • Has an intervention for substance or alcohol misuse been proposed? • Is seclusion or restraint necessary? • What level of physical security is needed? How should any further episodes of violence be managed? • Is the risk of violence imminent? • What antecedents are there to look out for? • Has a Care Programme Approach been implemented? • Has a Community Treatment Order been considered? • Has an assertive outreach approach been considered? • Has everyone from carers to professionals been adequately consulted and informed about the risks present and the interventions required? • Are they realistic in their expectations?

Source: Royal College of Psychiatrists (2016).

of both nature and degree of a disorder (despite the lack of reference to this in the MHA), how then should it be assessed? While a range of assessment tools is described, (Reddy, 2015), these do not appear to be widely used in clinical practice and other approaches are therefore needed. Amador and Kronengold (2004), suggest that insight has five different dimensions:

1. Awareness of having a mental illness.
2. Awareness of the consequences of mental illness.
3. Awareness of symptoms of mental disorder
4. Attribution of symptoms to a mental disorder
5. Awareness of the effects of medication.

Applying this model may suggest that failure to satisfy all five limbs may be regarded as a lack of insight, noting that this model is not validated and only serves as a guide. Reddy (2015) suggests that the outcome of assessment of insight may be any of:

1. Complete denial of illness.
2. Slight awareness of being sick and needing help but denying it at the same time.
3. Awareness of being sick but blaming it on others or external events.
4. Intellectual insight.
5. True emotional insight

It would seem inaccurate to deem an individual as lacking capacity unless a systematic assessment has been undertaken using a validated insight assessment tool or the Amador and

Kronengold (2004) model described above. Use of terms such as "partial insight" need clarification. Insight may well fluctuate and may never have been present – here, details about an individual's baseline beliefs and function are needed, although it may not always be possible to obtain satisfactory evidence about this. In such situations, careful consideration of the clinical evidence and conducting thorough fact finding will guide decision making.

Appropriate Medical Treatment

This is a feature of treatment sections such as section 3, with medical treatment specifically defined in the MHA:

> medical treatment includes nursing, psychological intervention and specialist mental health habilitation, rehabilitation and care.
>
> (MHA 2007, s145)

Appropriate medical treatment is defined in the MHA thus:
"For the purposes of this Part of this Act, it is appropriate for treatment to be given to a patient if the treatment is appropriate in his case, taking into account the nature and degree of the mental disorder from which he is suffering and all other circumstances of his case", (MHA 2007, s 64(3). The purpose of medical treatment is also defined in the MHA:

> Any reference in this Act to medical treatment, in relation to mental disorder, shall be construed as a reference to medical treatment the purpose of which is to alleviate, or prevent a worsening of, the disorder or one or more of its symptoms or manifestations.
>
> (MHA, 2007, s 145(4))

It is therefore apparent that appropriate medical treatment encompasses a wide range of potential interventions, and has been considered in case law (Curtice, 2009, 2024). Phull and Bartlett (2012), suggesting that the definition of appropriate medical treatment needs, while vague, requires treatment consideration on an individual basis. They suggest that the following questions be considered when determining what constitutes appropriate medical treatment:

- What precisely is the treatment that can be provided and what is its purpose?
- Is the treatment actually available?
- What discernible benefit will it have for the patient? (This does not mean a cure is certain; it does mean that there is a reasonable likelihood that treatment will result in significantly better outcomes than non-treatment.)
- Are there adverse effects of the treatment that outweigh the benefits?
- Are the benefits related to the patient's mental disorder (either its symptoms or manifestations), or to some unrelated problem?

Conclusion

This chapter has briefly considered the key concepts of mental disorder and statutory legal aspects of mental disorder namely: nature, degree, and risks. It has also included a discussion about insight, noting that risk is not formally defined in the MHA, nor is insight mentioned there. Mental disorder remains complex and difficult to define and relies on elicitation of symptoms using structured approaches, with specific criteria for detention, all of which need to be met for someone to be detained. It is suggested that in all tribunals, understanding and consideration of definitions be used where they exist, that risks be considered in relation to the factors described in the Royal College of Psychiatrists Guidance (Table 1.4), that appropriate treatment be considered in relation to the questions formulated by Phull and Bartlett (2012), and that where insight is deemed lacking, the model proposed by Amador and Kronengold (2004), be applied. Overall, adopting robust approaches as described in this chapter as well as considering the advice contained in the MHA Code of Practice will assist the tribunal in making robust findings of fact, and thus achieving the overriding objective of enabling the tribunal to deal with cases fairly and justly.

References

Amador XF and Kronengold H (2004) Understanding and assessing insight, in Amador XF and David A (eds) *Insight and Psychosis: Awareness of Illness in Schizophrenia and Related Disorders* (2nd edn). Oxford: Oxford University Press.

Bolton J (2008) *What is Mental Disorder? An Essay in Philosophy, Science and Values*. Oxford: Oxford University Press.

Curtice MJR (2009) Medical treatment under Part IV of the Mental Health Act 1983 and the Human Rights Act 1998: review of Article 3 and 8 case law. *Psychiatric Bulletin*, 33(3): 111–115.

Curtice M (2024) The interface between the Mental Health Act and Mental Capacity Act: physical health treatment. *BJPsych Advance*, 2024: 1–9. doi:10.1192/bja.2023.66

Department of Health (2009) *Best Practice in Managing Risk Principles and Evidence for Best Practice in the Assessment and Management of Risk to Self and Others in Mental Health Services*. London: Department of Health.

de Vries M and Bijlsma J (2022) The elusive concept of dangerousness: the state of the art in criminal legal theory and the necessity of further research. *Criminal Justice Ethics*, 41(2): 142–166.

Dixon LB, Holoshitz Y and Nossel I (2016) Treatment engagement of individuals experiencing mental illness: review and update. *World Psychiatry*, 15: 13–20.

Drapeau A, Marchand A and Beaulieu-Prévost D (2012) Epidemiology of psychological distress, in L'Abate L (ed) *Mental Illnesses–Understanding, Prediction and Control*. Rijeka, Croatia: InTech.

Fanning J (2016) Continuities of risk in the era of the mental capacity act. *Medical Law Review*, 24(3): 415–433.

Guidry-Grimes L (2019) Ethical complexities in assessing patients' insight. *Journal of Medical Ethics*, 45: 178–182.

Large MM, Ryan CJ, Nielssen OB and Hayes RA (2008) The danger of dangerousness: why we must remove the dangerousness criterion from our mental health acts. *Journal of Medical Ethics*, 34: 877–881.

Marková IS and Berrios GE (1992) The meaning of insight in clinical psychiatry. *British Journal of Psychiatry*, 160(6): 850–860.

Matarazzo JD (1978) The interview: its reliability and validity in psychiatric diagnosis, in Wolman BB (ed) *Clinical Diagnosis of Mental Disorders*. Boston, MA: Springer.

Mental Health Act (2007). Legislation.gov.uk

Phull J and Bartlett P (2012) 'Appropriate' medical treatment: what's in a word? *Medicine. Science and the Law*, 52(2): 71–74.

Reddy MS (2015) Insight and psychosis. *Indian Journal of Psychological Medicine*, 37: 257–260.

Royal College of Psychiatrists (2016) *Good Practice Guide: Assessment and Management of Risk to Others*. London: Royal College of Psychiatrists.

Schaafsma SM, Pfaff DW, Spunt RP and Adolphs R (2015) Deconstructing and reconstructing theory of mind. *Trends Cognitive Science*, 19(2): 65–72.

Szasz T (1961) *The Myth of Mental Illness*. London: Martin Secker & Warburg.

Tait G (2010) Some problems with the meaning of 'disorder', in Tait G (ed) *Philosophy, Behaviour Disorders, and the School*. Leiden: Brill.

Varga S. (2015) *Naturalism, Interpretation, and Mental Disorder.* Oxford: Oxford University Press.

Wakefield JC and First MB (2013) Clarifying the boundary between normality and disorder: a fundamental conceptual challenge for psychiatry. *Canadian Journal of Psychiatry*, 58(11): 603–605.

Wand T (2011) Investigating the evidence for the effectiveness of risk assessment in mental health care. *Issues in Mental Health Nursing*, 33(1): 2–7.

Wheeler R and Ruck Keene A (2022) Compulsory treatment of physical illness under MHA 1983. *Journal of Medical Ethics*, 48(11): 821–824.

WHO (2022) *Mental Disorders.* [online] Available at: www.who.int/news-room/fact-sheets/detail/mental-disorders (accessed 29 August 2024).

CASES CITED

Attia v British Gas [1998] Q.B. 304

B v Croydon Health Authority [1995] 1 All E.R. 683):

R. (on the application of B) v Ashworth Hospital Authority [2005] UKHL 20; [2005] 2 All E.R.

R v Deighton [2005] EWCA Crim 3131

R v Mental Health Review Tribunal for the South Thames Region Ex p. Smith [1999] C.O.D.

R (Smith) v MHRT South Thames Region (1998) EWHC Admin 832

R. v North West London Mental Health NHS Trust Ex p. Stewart (1996) 39 B.M.L.R. 105

St George's Healthcare NHS Trust v S [1988] 3 All E.R. 673

Smirek v Williams [2002] M.H.L.R. 38148

Winterwerp v Netherlands (1979) E.H.R.R. 387

FURTHER READING

MHA Code of Practice (Department of Health (2015) *Reference Guide to the Mental Health Act.* Norwich: The Stationery Office)

This is the definitive guide as to how to interpret and apply the MHA and contains, among others, a chapter relating to tribunal process and a plethora of other practical information.

Oyebode F (2022) *Sims' Symptoms in the Mind: Textbook of Descriptive Psychopathology* (7th edn). Amsterdam: Elsevier.

This is the 7th edition of a classic book that details potential symptoms of mental disorder with multiple chapters and clear explanations. It is well-written and easy to read and is a useful reference source, covering a wide range of background topics and presentations.

Burns T (2006) *Psychiatry: A Short Introduction.* Oxford: Oxford University Press.

This provides a precise, readable presentation of what psychiatry is and includes a discussion of the history of psychiatry as well as its limitations.

2 The Role of Medication in Treatment

John S Watts

Introduction

This chapter will open with a discussion of the history of medication use in mental health, followed by an explanation of how drugs are administered. After this, there is some information given regarding naming conventions, prescribing indications, and classification. Suggestions for the presentation of written and oral evidence follows this, with a consideration of the non-disclosure of information, before some concluding comments are made. The content of this chapter is founded upon the author's experience of both presenting evidence to the hearing panel as a medical witness and receiving that evidence as a medical member of the tribunal hearing panel. Much of what is discussed and explored is the author's opinion, and not official advice or guidance. However, it is important to note that there is no substitute for direct experience, and observations of tribunal hearings, and evidence gathering is encouraged before assuming the "hot seat" and presenting written or oral evidence to the panel members. The current process for observing hearings is less involved than in the recent past, but still requires some advance planning. The patient needs to be asked to consent to the observer's attendance, and it is good practice to involve the patient's representative in this process, as they will be asked during the hearing for permission or objections by the tribunal. The tribunal will also need to consent to the request, and it is wise to do this ahead of the hearing by contacting it through the trust's Mental Health Act office or equivalent. In addition, the experience of being part of a mock or practice hearing, either as part of a course or study module, or arranged informally with colleagues with prior tribunal experience, is a worthwhile exercise in exposure and anxiety management. Such practice can also help the witness to hone the necessary skills required when giving evidence. Although some inexperienced witnesses may fear, or even dread hearing participation, but preparation and practice can mitigate these feelings, and it is not unusual for many to actually enjoy the experience. It is an opportunity to demonstrate an understanding of the patient and their risks, to discuss treatment and management, and to explore some of the issues at the interface of the law and medicine.

A Brief History of Medication Use in Mental Health

Psychotropic medication, that is, medication used to treat and alleviate the symptoms of psychiatric illnesses and disorders, has a long history of use in psychiatry and in the treatment of mental illnesses and disorders. The Mental Health Act makes reference to "Mental Disorders" but does not define this. The code of practice makes some attempts by giving examples, but a legal definition remains somewhat elusive, (Department of Health, 2015). In the author's

DOI: 10.4324/9781003635543-3

experience, the terms "psychiatric illness", "psychiatric disorder", "mental illness", and "mental disorder" are often used interchangeably and synonymously.

An example of a medicine that has been used for decades in psychiatry is lithium. Lithium is a metal element and is normally administered orally to the patient as a tablet containing the metal salt such as lithium carbonate or lithium citrate. Lithium has been in use from the 1940s (and probably before) for the treatment of mania, and chlorpromazine from the 1950s (Harrison et al, 2018, p 711). The trade name for chlorpromazine, when it was first introduced, was "Largactil", a nod to the wide range of actions it has on multiple neurotransmitter systems.

Medication forms an important part of the management of many mental illnesses and conditions, and thus it is vital that the reasons for prescribing, plus the response, compliance of the patient, and effectiveness of the treatment is presented as evidence to the tribunal. Treatment response forms a part of the nature of the mental disorder and will also form part of the evidence when discussing the degree.

Methods of Medication Administration

Most of the medications used in mental health treatment are given orally. The patient either has to swallow a tablet or capsule, or drink the drug in liquid form, in order for it to be absorbed into the bloodstream. There are obviously advantages to giving medication orally, such as convenience, shelf life (how long the medication can be kept without deterioration), and ease of use (for the patient to take themselves). Liquid medication can also be given via naso-gastric tube, sometimes of relevance in patients with eating disorders, and via the rectum, an example being diazepam (Valium®). The types of medications given orally include medications that act immediately, for example the methylphenidate formulation branded Ritalin®, or slow or sustained release, such as the methylphenidate formulation branded Concerta XL®. Medications given orally are absorbed into the blood stream (mostly the plasma) through the digestive system, so can be affected by food and drink, and usually take 30–60 minutes minimum to start to exert their effects. Absorption of orally-administered drugs will also be affected in patients with digestion issues, an example being patients with chronic alcohol dependence. Examples of drugs given orally include antidepressants such as sertraline and agomelatine, antipsychotics such as aripiprazole and lurasidone, and mood stabilisers such as sodium valproate and lithium, to name but a few.

Drugs can also be given as injections. These can be given intramuscularly (IM, commonly given in the gluteal muscle in the buttock, the ventro gluteal muscle or the deltoid muscle in the shoulder), subcutaneously (SC, just under the skin), intradermally (a little deeper under the skin) or intravenously (IV, directly into a vein, normally in the arm). The advantage of this method is that it is an option when a patient cannot swallow, or when they are refusing the treatment and it has to be given. Disadvantages include discomfort or pain with administration, privacy and dignity associated with exposure of injection sites and the potential for soft tissue damage. Examples of injectable agents include the benzodiazepine lorazepam, the sedative antihistamine promethazine, and the antipsychotic olanzapine. IM is often the mode used during rapid tranquilisation, due to the slightly quicker absorption compared with orally administered agents, and the ability to administer to a resisting patient being held under physical restraint. It is also used when medications are denatured (and hence rendered ineffective) by digestive enzymes, so cannot be taken orally (an example outside of mental health treatment is insulin being given for type 1 diabetes).

Another group of drugs given as injections are the depot medications, which are mostly used in the mental health field in the treatment of chronic schizophrenia and other psychoses. These are usually active drugs combined with an oil, resulting in a formulation that releases the drug very slowly. They are a very useful mode of drug delivery, as they can be given less frequently than oral medications and are given in the buttock or shoulder. They are mostly used when medication compliance is an issue, but sometimes are chosen by the patient for convenience reasons. The frequency of injections can vary from 2 weeks up to every 6 months. Because of their slow duration of action, they take a very long time to get to a steady state in the blood (months compared with days for oral medications), and if the patient experiences adverse effects, there is no way to withdraw the drug. Because of this issue with adverse effects, other medications may need to be added to the patient's treatment regime to try to manage these effects whilst waiting for the levels of the drug in the blood to reduce. Examples of depots include zuclopentixol, (Clopixol®), paliperidone and olanzapine.

Less common methods of psychiatric drug administration also exist. For example, esketamine, (Spravato®), can be used in depressive disorders as a nasal spray, and nicotine replacement therapy can be administered as a skin patch (transdermal), a sublingual tablet (under the tongue), a chewing gum, an inhalator, and a nasal spray.

Relevance of Medication Treatment in Mental Health Tribunals

Medication, or physical treatment, is an important part of the management of many psychiatric disorders as discussed above, and thus will need to form part of the written and oral evidence presented to the tribunal. Physical treatments for mental disorders include not just medication, but also electro-convulsive therapy (ECT), transcranial magnetic stimulation (TMS), and surgical interventions ("psychosurgery").

Although the assumption of this chapter is that the readership will consist of experienced mental health practitioners, including those with expertise in prescribing in the mental health field, it may be useful to start with a general discussion of different types of medication, their use, and examples of some notable adverse effects. The term "adverse effects" is used here in preference to the term "side effects", as it more accurately portrays the negative or unintended actions of a drug on the human body.

Medication Naming Conventions and Indications for Use

It is worthwhile taking a brief detour into the drug development world at this point, before discussing medication examples in more detail, in order to illustrate why most medications have two or more names. Almost all psychotropics are initially designated by a pharmaceutical company or university research department by a series of letters and numbers. These are usually not memorable. Once a drug candidate molecule shows promise in treating the intended illness or disorder, the researchers and developers, or others in the institution, will produce a generic, or official name for the molecule. It is only at the point of registration with a country's medicines regulatory authority that a brand name will be allocated. The generic name may be more memorable than the previously designated letters and numbers, but the author has often pondered whether it is sometimes a deliberate ploy by pharmaceutical companies to create a difficult to pronounce or recall generic name, so that the brand name is recalled preferentially. In the UK, the medicines regulatory authority is the Medicines and Healthcare products Regulatory Agency, (MHRA).

As an example of this naming convention, a recent Pfizer drug used for smoking cessation started life as CP 526,555 (not easily memorable); it then gained the generic name varenicline tartrate (somewhat easier to remember, but maybe not to pronounce) when it was available in the UK to be prescribed, and started to be marketed, it gained the brand name Champix®, or Chantix® in other countries, (much easier to recall and repeat), (National Library of Medicine, 2010).

Once the patent on a drug expires, other companies are entitled to then produce their own versions of the medicine, and to fabricate their own trade name. The new company has to demonstrate to the regulatory authority that their version of the drug is the same active compound as the one they are copying. This is normally achieved by conducting so-called "non-inferiority" studies which are then submitted to the medicines regulatory authority (U.S. Food and Drug Administration, 2016). An example of this would be the long-acting version of the stimulant Concerta XL®. The generic name of the drug is methylphenidate, and it was originally marketed as Concerta XL® by the company Janssen-Cilag. Currently in the UK it is available as Delmosart® (Accord-UK), Matoride XL® (Sandoz), Xaggitin XL® (Ethypharm) and Xenidate XL® (Viatris UK Healthcare). Thus the reader can see that one compound may have many different names but contain the same active ingredient and have the same mode of action. It can also be appreciated why it is important to use the generic name where possible and appropriate.

Turning now to a discussion of indications for medicines, pharmaceutical companies will need to apply to a country's medicines regulatory authority for authorisation to market a medication, and for it to be available to be prescribed. In order for this authorisation to be granted, evidence will need to be presented by the company to the regulatory authority for it to be assessed and evaluated. This may include evidence from computer models, animal studies, first in human safety trials, trials showing the efficacy in the target patient population, safety data, information on the composition of the active ingredient and the excipients, and the stability of the preparation. Excipients are the "extra bits" that make up the whole tablet or preparation, in addition to the active ingredient, and can include substances such as starch, lactose, and phosphates (European Medicines Agency, 2021). Once the regulatory authority is satisfied with the evidence, and they are confident the medicine is safe enough for use in the patient population, the preparation will be authorised for use, or more correctly a marketing authorisation will be granted, and the indication, or indications for use will be specified. This will be the licensed indication.

However, medications can often show efficacy and promise in other indications in addition to the originally licensed ones. Therefore, medications are often prescribed for conditions and symptoms that are not authorised in advance by the regulatory authority. This does not mean that the medication does not work as well for the unlicensed indication as for the licensed indication, rather that the regulatory authority has not reviewed or accepted study or trial evidence that has been submitted to them by the pharmaceutical company, and therefore a marketing authorisation cannot be considered and then granted. Thus, a medicine can be used for a licensed indication, such as the use of fluoxetine for depression, or for an off-label indication, one that it does not have a license or marketing authorisation for, such as the use of fluoxetine for menstrual symptoms.

Care must be taken when using the terms "off-label" and "unlicensed" in a discussion regarding the use of medicines for particular disorders. Many people use the terms interchangeably, and thus they may misunderstand their definitions. "Off-label" is the term used when a medicine with a marketing authorisation for one disorder is prescribed for another disorder or indication for which it does not have a marketing authorisation. In this context, "label" is being used as a synonym for "licensed indication". The term "unlicensed" is used when is medicine is prescribed for an indication for which there is no marketing authorisation, and the medicine does not have an authorisation for any other indication in that country, (Aronson and Ferner, 2017). It may be important for the tribunal to be informed whether the medication is being used for a licensed indication, or if it is being used off-label or for unlicensed use.

Classification of Psychotropic Medicines

Psychotropic medications can be grouped together in many different ways. In the author's opinion, the most logical method is to classify them according to their chief, licensed or original intended mode of action: antipsychotics, antidepressants, mood stabilisers, anxiolytics, hypnotics, and psychostimulants, (Harrison et al., 2018, p719). Please see the box for examples of members of each group, some adverse effects, and common indications for use. For up-to-date information on UK prescribed drugs, the interested reader is directed to the current version of the British National Formulary (British National Formulary, 2024), and the summaries of product characteristics available for free online, (Electronic Medicines Compendium, 2024).

Antipsychotics include so-called first-generation compounds such as chlorpromazine and haloperidol, and second-generation drugs such as aripiprazole and clozapine. An older method of classifying antipsychotics proposed splitting them into "typicals" and "atypicals", focusing on their modes of action and adverse effects. Typical antipsychotics tended to produce so-called extra-pyramidal adverse effects, and atypicals were considered to be relatively free of these. However, this system was considered too simplistic, and there were many overlaps between the two groups, and so it was mostly abandoned. However, it is not unusual to hear these medicines still being referred to in those terms. Antipsychotics were originally used to treat psychotic illnesses such as schizophrenia and mania. Since their first use, they have also shown efficacy in other disorders, such as treatment resistant mood disorders and personality disorders. Adverse effects of first-generation antipsychotics include extra pyramidal adverse effects such as tremor, muscle or limb rigidity and parkinsonism, and often require separate medication treatments to help manage these symptoms, such as the anticholinergic compound procyclidine. Adverse effects of the second-generation antipsychotics include weight gain, metabolic effects, and electro-cardiogram (ECG) changes.

   Antidepressants include older medications such as amitriptyline and lofepramine, and newer entities such as fluoxetine and mirtazapine. Unsurprisingly, they were originally used to treat mood disorders such as depression, but are also now prescribed for anxiety disorders, obsessive compulsive disorders, and sometimes for trauma and sleep issues. Adverse effects can include sedation, weight gain, increased suicidal thoughts, and ECG abnormalities.

   Mood stabilisers include antiepileptics such as lamotrigine and sodium valproate, lithium salts, and some antipsychotics. Their main use in mental health is in the treatment of bipolar disorder and mania, but they are also used for augmentation of treatment in depression, especially when it is treatment resistant. When a drug is used for augmentation, it is added to the current treatment. Adverse effects include weight gain and sedation, and effects on foetal development.

   Anxiolytics (from Greek, literally cutting anxiety) are used primarily to treat anxiety disorders, but they can also be used for short-term calming and tranquilisation.

They are often a key component of rapid tranquilisation protocols, used when a patient requires emergency calming when very distressed and agitated, alongside antipsychotics. Members of this group include the barbiturates such as phenobarbitone (barbiturates are almost never prescribed for this indication now due to their toxicity in overdose), the benzodiazepines such as diazepam, and buspirone. Adverse effects include sedation and respiratory rate depression, and most carry a risk of tolerance and dependence.

Hypnotics (also from Greek meaning to cause sleep) are used to aid sleep initiation and duration and include the benzodiazepines and "Z" drugs such as zopiclone and zolplidem (officially the "Z" drugs are termed cyclopyrrolones, but they are rarely referred to as such for obvious reasons). Adverse effects are similar to the anxiolytics, and there are particular concerns around tolerance and dependence.

Psychostimulants, more usually termed 'stimulants', are used to treat Attention Deficit Hyperactivity Disorder (ADHD, sometimes referred to as Hyperkinetic Disorder) and narcolepsy. Members include methylphenidate and dexamfetamine. Adverse effects include appetite suppression, growth velocity reduction, and blood pressure issues.

Others: These drugs do not fit neatly in the above classification and include the non-stimulant ADHD treatments atomoxetine and guanfacine, anticholinergic drugs such as procyclidine used to manage antipsychotic extra-pyramidal adverse effects and short-term distress alleviators such as the antihistamine promethazine.

Presenting the Evidence to the Tribunal Panel

Written Evidence

There now follow some comments and suggestions regarding the presentation of written evidence to the tribunal. The authors of reports for the tribunal should consult the Practice Direction for Statements and Reports, which outlines the minimum information required in reports (tribunals Judiciary, 2013). The report writers are strongly advised to avail themselves of a copy of this document, and to follow the requirements closely. However, the information asked for by the Practice Direction is often not sufficient to convey all the important and relevant information regarding the patient and the plans to the tribunal, and the report authors are encouraged not to feel constrained by the information requested. There is also the option of providing other reports and written evidence to the tribunal as an addendum or addenda. For instance, copies of multi-agency meeting minutes, psychiatric reports, Second Opinion Appointed Doctor (SOAD) reports and certificates, and details of section 117 planning meetings can often be useful to the panel and will add extra detail to the statutory reports. The SOAD will provide a report and certificate if a patient is not consenting to, or is unable to consent to medication administration following a three month period of taking the medication whilst being detained in hospital (Care Quality Commission, 2024). The written evidence needs to be presented in clear and understandable English, with any jargon or acronyms explained or spelled out the first time they are used. Although the tribunal has its own medical expertise, it is good practice to write the reports without assuming a detailed knowledge of psychiatric terminology and experience of psychopharmacology in the reader. It is also worth noting that the patient is likely to read the report, usually with the support of their representative. Although most tribunal members will be comfortable in using Latin terminology such as prn (pro re nata, Latin for 'as required', when used with reference to medication, it applies to drugs that are not prescribed for regular administration, and are thus used when they are needed), it does not cost much to translate and explain. Likewise, when introducing medicine names, it is wise to use the generic name (please see discussion above for details of this) and to include some explanatory text, such as: "the patient was started on the oral antipsychotic olanzapine with the aim of treating the auditory hallucinations", which again should facilitate the non-expert's fluid intake of information.

All pages need to be numbered, as should the paragraphs. The report needs to be written specifically for the hearing, and although the Practice Direction advises against copying and pasting from previous reports, it is often advice that is ignored. When this does occur, the report author is advised to read each passage carefully, ensuring that the style and tone fits in with the whole report. Special attention needs to be paid to dates and times. For instance, the phrase 'was taking olanzapine two years ago' may have been accurate when used in a report five years previously but becomes incorrect if recycled without updating in a more recent report.

Oral Evidence

With regards to presentation of the oral evidence, the usual practice of the tribunal during the hearing is for the medical member of the panel to commence with asking questions of the RC or their representative. This often starts with a focus on the evidence for the statutory criteria for detention and applies to the evidence being presented that day. It is likely, therefore, that the first oral discussion of medication will take place when appropriate treatment is explored, noting that this will not be the case for some hearings, such as for section 2. The witness will sometimes be asked to confirm they continue to agree with the contents of the report submitted to the panel beforehand, and whether they have any substantive updates. If the witness is not the report author, they may be asked if they agree with the report and its opinions, and if not, why not. This may not be due to variance in professional opinion, as the presentation or degree of the patient's mental disorder may have changed since the report was written. Responses to questions should be addressed to the panel, which is obviously only relevant in face-to-face hearings.

It is acceptable to ask for time to confirm an answer or the origin of evidence, and a short adjournment could be requested if vital information needs to be checked, and this is not immediately available. Evidence should be given in a clear voice and should be relevant to the question that prompts it. Often the judge will start by asking the medical witness to confirm which statutory criteria are being relied upon on the day of the hearing and will expect "yes" or "no" responses. Please bear in mind that the judge themselves will be producing a written record of the hearing, so please be mindful of the speed of your delivery of information, which will be greatly appreciated. Again, as with written evidence, please explain any jargon that is used, and be willing to provide evidence for a particular medicine choice if this is outside of current guidelines or usual practice.

Information That is Required and Helpful for the Tribunal

The Practice Direction includes requirements for reports regarding patients in hospital and in the community, (Tribunals Judiciary, 2013). Medication is mentioned on six occasions, the first in the requirements for the inpatient responsible clinician report (Tribunals Judiciary, 2013, p 4). The report author needs to address the patient's understanding of the medication, their current compliance with it, and the "future willingness" to continue to take prescribed medication. It will therefore be important for the tribunal to be presented with evidence of the patient's capacity (if over 16), or Gillick competence (if under 16 years) to consent to the psychotropic medication being given, which includes whether the patient understands the rationale for the treatment and medicine choice (British and Irish Legal Information Institute, 1985). It is unlikely but possible that details of the assessment of Mental Capacity or competence will be required, but it would be wise to be able to provide the date of the last assessment of that understanding, and also whether section 58 of the mental health act is engaged, the so-called three-month rule, (Department of Health, 2015). If the patient is being treated under a T2 or T3 certificate, or a CTO11 or CTO12 form, then this needs to be mentioned, including the dates of authorisation, and by whom. If a patient lacks the capacity or competence to consent to medication administration, or if they have that ability but are declining to take the prescribed medicines, and they fulfil the section 58 criteria but have not been seen by a SOAD, then the tribunal may require further explanation and justification. Treatments under the Act need to be lawful.

With regards to compliance, nurses are often better placed than prescribers to supply detailed and nuanced information regarding the patient's co-operation with the treatment regime. However, there is no reason why this detailed information cannot be obtained from colleagues and included in reports before the hearing. It may also be important to state negatives where this is relevant. For example, in a patient who has a history of stock-piling medication for future suicide attempts, the report could state, "the patient has been taking their oral antidepressant mirtazapine regularly, with no evidence of concealing the tablets in their mouth, and no evidence of hoarding any tablets".

Details are important, as well as the context for any comments. Inpatient wards, care homes and teams often have different rules and procedures for the different possible levels of medication administration, and the tribunal may not be aware of your local practice. If a patient is permitted to self-administer or take their own medication, this is useful and relevant evidence for the tribunal to receive. For instance, is the patient given a dosette box, (a tablet holding box with compartments showing times and days of administration), at the beginning of the week or month, or do they have to request that the medication is dispensed and given to them? At the very least, it is good practice to discuss whether the patient requires prompting to take medication, whether they will seek out nursing or care staff to administer, whether there is any resistance by the patient to taking the medication, or any negative communication or behaviour responses when the drug is administered.

As part of any discussion of medication, either verbally or in written form, some discussion of adverse effects would be expected. Aside from any direct morbidity induced by such effects (for example the metabolic effects of olanzapine), the impact on compliance, or future willingness to continue, would be important for the tribunal to explore when evidence is given. If rating scales have been used to quantify and monitor adverse effects, these should be included in the report. It is also important to draw a distinction between observed effects, and those reported by the patient (often these are referred to as symptoms and signs: symptoms are reported by the patient, signs are observed by the professional). It is possible that the patient is reporting adverse effects that are not observed by others, or the opposite could be true.

The report writer, and hearing witness, also needs to address what appropriate treatment is available (when this is relevant to the current detention), of which medication may well form a significant part. Both of these points will be required in the community/community treatment order (CTO) RC report, in the RC report for conditionally discharged patients, and the nursing report. The tribunal needs to take evidence on the availability of appropriate treatment when considering the statutory criteria in detentions using sections 3, 17A, 36, 37, and 47, and medication often forms a part of this criterion. However, even in detentions not including appropriate treatment as a statutory criterion, (namely section 2 and guardianship), it is likely this type of information will still be required and requested. Appropriate treatment is not defined in the Act, but there is a chapter in the Code devoted to the subject (Department of Health, 2015, Chapter 23). Medical treatment is:

… for the purpose of alleviating, or preventing a worsening of, a mental disorder or one or more of its symptoms or manifestations', and that 'Purpose is not the same as likelihood.'

(Department of Health, 2015, p 246)

The term "medical treatment" is used here in the legal sense, and includes "nursing, psychological intervention and … habilitation, rehabilitation and care", and includes medication, (Department of Health, 2015, p 248). This is a much wider definition than most would use for clinical contexts, and it is worth noting that clinical and legal words may look the same, but their meanings and definitions are often not.

For treatment to be accepted as appropriate, the code of practice states that the nature and degree of the disorder must be considered, as well as assessing the purpose, (Department of Health, 2015, p 247). The chapter in the code is entitled, 'The appropriate medical treatment test', thus implying that a judgement needs to be passed on whether the treatment in question warrants the term 'appropriate', (Department of Health, 2015, p246). The tribunal has its own special medical expertise, namely an experienced psychiatrist sitting as the medical member, and other panel members will often have knowledge and skills relevant to psychotropic medication use, but for that expertise to be utilised, the medical evidence needs to be sufficient, clear and relevant in order for the tribunal to decide if the appropriate treatment criterion is met for detention. It is good practice to mention the form of the medication, such as tablet, liquid or injection, (please see the discussion above).

Non-disclosure of Information

Before concluding this chapter, a special mention will be made for the rules and circumstances concerning the non-disclosure of information to the patient. The procedure for this is covered in the tribunal procedure rules, and it is important for report writers and witnesses to be aware of the scope and limits to this process, (Tribunals Judiciary, 2008). It is of particular relevance to the subject matter of this chapter, as there are instances where a clinical team need to administer medication to a patient "in a disguised format" as the patient is refusing to take the medication, they lack capacity or competence, and the medication is essential, (Care Quality Commission, 2022).

Although the clinical threshold for withholding this information from patients is high, it is fair to say that within the arena of a tribunal that threshold is even higher. The Tribunal not only has to consider that the patient learning would "likely cause that person or some other person serious harm", but that it is in the interest of justice and is proportionate to hide from the patient (Tribunals Judiciary, 2008, p 11). It is a general principle in law that it is only fair that a patient is aware of all the evidence before the court, or in this case, the tribunal, so the reader can appreciate that there has to be sufficient evidence of the harm to the patient in order to override this maxim.

The process for asking the tribunal to not disclose information is to submit this information separately from any reports, and to mark it very clearly that it is not to be disclosed to the patient without the tribunal's consent. It is important to avoid making any direct or indirect references in the reports to this additional information being in existence. The tribunal will then usually consider the request as a preliminary matter before the hearing commences. It is not unusual for the tribunal to disagree with the request and allow the disclosure of the information to the patient. Therefore, report writers and witnesses are advised to consider with the clinical team how to deal with the situation whereby the patient learns of the covert administration of their medication, and hence be able to formulate a plan moving forward.

Conclusion

One of the functions of the Mental Health Tribunal is to be a safeguard against unwarranted and unlawful detentions and use of the Mental Health Act. In order for the tribunal to perform this function, it needs good quality evidence. This chapter has attempted to provide some guidance and suggestions as to how the evidence regarding medication and drug treatment can fulfil this aim. Although the hearing panel members sit in a legal arena, on a similar footing to a court of law, professionals need not fear their attendance and participation. Preparation is a key aspect in achieving this aim, both in terms of gathering the information for the report and the hearing, and with respect to being confident as an orator and verbal witness. Each hearing will be different from the last, but all have the same basic format and aims. Applying the skills and knowledge obtained from training courses, practice, observations and from ingesting this chapter should stand the reader in good stead for future hearing performances.

References and Further Reading

Aronson JK and Ferner RE, 2017. Unlicensed and off-label uses of medicines: definitions and clarification of terminology. *British Journal of Clinical Pharmacology* 83: 2615–2625.

British and Irish Legal Information Institute, 1985. *Gillick Respondent and West Norfolk and Wisbech Area Health Authority First Appellants and Department of Health and Social Care and Social Security Second Appellants* [online] Available at: www.bailii.org/uk/cases/UKHL/1985/7.html (accessed: 09 October 2024)

British National Formulary, 2024. [online] Available at: https://bnf.nice.org.uk/ (accessed: 09 October 2024)

Care Quality Commission, 2022. *Covert administration of medicines* [online] Available at: www.cqc.org.uk/guidance-providers/adult-social-care/covert-administration-medicines (accessed: 09 October 2024)

Care Quality Commission, 2024. *Request a SOAD (second opinion appointed doctor)* [online] Available at: www.cqc.org.uk/guidance-providers/nhs-trusts/second-opinion-appointed-doctors-soads (accessed: 09 October 2024).

Department of Health 2015. *Mental Health Act 1983: Code of Practice.* London: The Stationary Office.

Electronic Medicines Compendium, 2024. *Up to date, approved and regulated prescribing and patient information for licensed medicines* [online] Available at: www.medicines.org.uk/emc (accessed: 09 October 2024)

European Medicines Agency, 2021. *Excipients labelling* [online] Available at: www.ema.europa.eu/en/human-regulatory-overview/marketing-authorisation/product-information-requirements/excipients-labelling (accessed: 09 October 2024).

Harrison, P, Cowen, P, Burns, T and Fazel, M, 2018. *Shorter Oxford Textbook of Psychiatry.* 7th ed. Oxford: Oxford University Press.

National Library of Medicine, 2010. *National Center for Biotechnology Information* [online] Available at: https://classic.clinicaltrials.gov/ct2/show/NCT00594204 (accessed: 09 October 2024)

Tribunals Judiciary, 2008. The Tribunal Procedure (First-Tier Tribunal) (Health, Education and Social Care Chamber) Rules 2008 S.I. 2008 No. 2699 (L.16) [online] Available at: https://assets.publishing.service.gov.uk/media/663c9fa81c82a7597d4f333e/consolidated-FtT-HESCC-Rules.pdf (accessed: 09 October 2024)

Tribunals Judiciary, 2013. *Practice Direction. First-Tier Tribunal. Health Education and Social Care Chamber. Statements and Reports in Mental Health Cases.* [online] Available at: www.judiciary.uk/wp-content/uploads/2022/09/statements-in-mental-health-cases-hesc-28102013.pdf (accessed: 09 October 2024)

U.S. Food and Drug Administration, 2016. Non-Inferiority Clinical Trials to Establish Effectiveness - Guidance for Industry. Center for Drug Evaluation and Research (CDER) Center for Biologics Evaluation and Research (CBER), US.

3 Psychotherapeutic Treatment

Jane Roberts and Andy Cook

Introduction

The term psychotherapy refers to a variety of treatments that aim to help a person identify and change troubling emotions, thoughts, and behaviours. It can be delivered via a range of methods including talking, art, music, and drama; with talking being the most common, hence the term "talking therapies". Engagement in therapy can be one-to-one, in family groups or small network groups, or in groups that have specifically come together for the therapy. When seeking therapy as a member of the public one, has a great degree of autonomy, confidentiality, and choice in terms of therapist, modality of treatment, and goals for treatment. There is an astonishing variety of therapeutic approaches available with an estimated excess of 500 different types of psycho-therapy available 500 (Lilienfeld & Arkowitz, 2012). However, many common features can be established across therapeutic modalities, which will be discussed later in this chapter.

Those detained or subject to conditions under the Mental Health Act have much less autonomy, confidentiality, and choice associated with treatment. Treatment can be mandated or can be experienced as offered with a high degree of coercion. Services have a duty to protect the public as well as promote personal recovery, so treatment often has a dual purpose of reducing risk to self and others, and alleviating distress related to mental illness. Often the two go hand-in-hand in that treating mental health problems will have a positive impact on risk posed to self and/or others. Understanding the interplay between risk, mental health and the personal goals of the client is key in developing a treatment plan. Sharing of information between professionals is a key component of risk monitoring and management.

Is Psychological Treatment Indicated?

A psychological assessment is the ideal starting place, as beginning treatment without a robust understanding of the presenting issues may lead to ineffective treatment, disengagement, and wasted time and resources. The assessment should lead to an individualised formulation indicating the key targets for intervention and considerations for personalising intervention delivery, such as cognitive ability or neurodiversity. An assessment would usually use a com-bination of sources of information including historical reports, clinical interview, observation, psychometrics, structured clinical judgement tools, and standardised tests. The information gathered is then integrated using psychological theory to hypothesise about the nature and origin of the problems, explaining how an individual comes to present with a certain disorder or cir-cumstance at a particular point in time. Personal meaning is the integrating factor in a psycho-logical formulation, with the emphasis on what people have experienced, how they have coped, and what resources they have to build on for future functioning (Johnstone et al., 2018). It is

DOI: 10.4324/9781003635543-4

extremely beneficial for the service user to be fully involved in the assessment, and to be a partner in developing the goals and agreeing the methods for treatment. This is key to the formation of a strong therapeutic alliance, the importance of which is addressed in this chapter.

If there has not been a psychological assessment then it would be prudent to recommend this as a starting point. If there has been an assessment previously then this should give some indications of targets for intervention. It would be important to then consider whether any previous interventions have been offered and whether any progress has been made, and what remains outstanding as a treatment need. Treatment needs should also be considered in terms of whether they are necessary to be addressed prior to discharge from hospital to enhance safety, whether they can be addressed whilst living in the community under supervision, or whether they could be addressed to maximise quality of life but are not essential to address for discharge from hospital or supervision. For example, it is usually considered necessary to address risk or offending behaviour. Conversely, addressing childhood trauma impact is usually considered best undertaken when, or if, the individual wishes to do so, provided that some stabilisation work has taken place and associated risk behaviours have been addressed.

Understanding Psychotherapeutic Models

There are a broad range of psychological theories and models which inform how formulations might be framed and also how psychotherapeutic treatments are constructed. The theories, models, and associated interventions do not exist in a hierarchy of usefulness or accurateness. There is a metaphor that likens problems to a locked door: in order to get through the locked door some people just want the key, others will want to know who locked the door, others will want to know how the lock works, some will want to know who put the door there and shut it in the first place, and others may just want to bash the door down! Perhaps what is most important is to identify the agreed goal and to use an approach which is a good fit for both the therapist and client. There is much research that highlights the trusting therapeutic relationship as the most important factor contributing to change, identifying the relationship as at least as important, if not more important, than the treatment method, (e.g. Norcross, 2011; Norcross & Lambert, 2018), as this is what enables a boundaried and safe reflective learning space and the opportunity for a reparative relational experience.

Having an overview of the therapeutic models is probably helpful in understanding the formulation and the treatment being offered. There are too many psychotherapeutic models to do justice to the full range here, but we have focused on some of the most popular, commonly-used and researched therapies. It is acknowledged that this is a brief summary of psychological therapies and there are many more, with even more being developed. It is beyond the scope of this chapter to summarise all available psychological therapies, and it is noted that there are many specialist therapies that are not detailed here.

Psychoanalytic/Psychodynamic Therapies

Psychodynamic therapies originated from the work of Sigmund Freud and were subsequently developed by prominent figures such as Melanie Klein. The terms psychodynamic and psychoanalytic are often used interchangeably but psychoanalysis refers to a specific form of therapy delivered by a psychoanalyst (Levy, 2009). Psychodynamic theory emphasises the influence of unconscious thoughts, desires, and early childhood. Psychodynamic treatment is often long-term, intensive and does not lend itself to a manualised approach. As such, the NHS does not commonly offer it. However, it can be usefully applied to making sense of problematic presentations, using concepts such as unconscious defences or drives. Additionally, psycho-dynamic groupwork has an established theory base (Yalom & Leszcz, 2005) and there is evidence that psychotherapeutic groups can be effective in specific settings (see for example, Woods, 2014). Attachment theory, which theorises about the impact of our relationships with our caregivers on our current functioning, has grown out of psychodynamic ideas.

Mentalisation-based Treatment

Mentalisation-based treatment (MBT) was developed in the 1990s by Anthony Bateman and Peter Fonagy specifically for people with borderline personalities (Bateman & Fonagy, 2010). Mentalising is the ability to focus on and differentiate between your own emotional state of mind and that of others and understand how one's mental state influences behaviour. Mentalisation is a normal capacity that we all use in everyday life to understand ourselves, others, and interpersonal interactions. The ability is developed in the context of our early attachment relationships, and those who have faced childhood trauma and/or disrupted attachment relationships can find it more difficult to mentalise in certain situations than others. Enhancement of mentalisation and improved emotional regulation are at the core of MBT treatment. MBT is based in psychoanalysis, attachment theory, and acceptance. It is an evidence-based treatment for emotionally unstable or so-called borderline personality disorder (EUPD/BPD) and is included in the NICE Guideline for the treatment of BPD (National Institute for Clinical Excellence (NICE), 2009).

Cognitive Behavioural Therapy

Cognitive Behavioural Therapy (CBT) was developed by Aaron T. Beck in the 1960s and 70s, (Beck & Fleming, 2021). CBT focuses on the individual's thoughts, feelings, and behaviours, identifying how these influence each other. There is an established evidence base for cognitive behavioural therapy, although some critiques suggest that there is an evidence base because it is a type of therapy that is highly focused and structured, and therefore lends itself to being researched, (Cook, Schwartz & Kaslow, 2017). It is also a form of therapy that often has a relatively short and specified duration, which is favourable for NHS settings where very lengthy therapeutic interventions would be very costly. CBT has an established evidence base for use with problems such as anxiety and depression. There are also specific versions of CBT for application with psychosis (CBT for psychosis or CBTp), and for trauma (Trauma Focused CBT or TF-CBT). CBT tends to be a carefully structured therapy where each session has an agreed agenda, and "homework" is a key feature of the model. CBT is particularly recommended for depression and psychosis; it is in the NICE guidelines for both disorders (National Institute for Clinical Excellence (NICE), 2022; National Institute for Clinical Excellence (NICE), 2014).

Third Wave CBT

"Third wave CBT" methods were developed to build on the CBT model, but to be more "focused on the *function* of cognition and emotion, over and above their form *per se*", (Hayes et al., 2021), looking at the relationship of the person to their experience. These are seen as process-oriented models. There are various different models of third wave therapies and they often involve concepts such as "acceptance, mindfulness, cognitive defusion, dialectics, values, spirituality, and relationship" (Hayes, 2004, p640). Examples of third wave CBT methods are Schema Therapy, Acceptance and Commitment Therapy (ACT), and Dialectical Behaviour Therapy (DBT).

Schema Therapy

Schema therapy (Young et al., 2003) was developed by Jeffrey Young in the late 1980s and early 1990s as a treatment for complex psychological problems. It is a longer-length intervention and is based on the theory that there are universal childhood needs (such as to be loved and have a secure attachment) and for some people these needs are not met, and that can at times result in Early Maladaptive Schemas developing. These schemas may have been initially adaptive in protecting the child psychologically from the harm or neglect as a child, but they are unhelpfully perpetuated through adulthood. The person develops coping modes based on flight, fight, or freeze from those schemas. For example, a person who was abused as a child may develop a mistrust/abuse schema, such that they anticipate mistrust or abuse from others and act accordingly. This may protect them as a child when the danger is still present. However, over the years this anticipation of mistrust/abuse may cause them to avoid relationships, or be hostile to partners, perhaps to attack partners before the anticipated harm can be inflicted. Schema therapy aims to heal the schemas. Schema therapy can be seen as an appropriate therapy option for people with entrenched personality problems who may struggle to benefit from "traditional" CBT (de Klerk et al., 2017), with evidence supporting its application for complex problems such as Borderline Personality Disorder, and in this instance, the optimal delivery is a combination of individual and group therapy (Arntz et al., 2022).

Dialectical Behaviour Therapy

Dialectical Behaviour Therapy (DBT) (Linehan, 1993) was developed by Marsha Linehan in the early 1990s to help chronically suicidal people, and was adapted over time to meet the needs of people who present with borderline personality disorder (BPD). It was the first treatment for BPD to demonstrate its efficacy in a Randomised Controlled Trial (Swales, 2009). It is a behavioural therapy and aims to identify and reinforce positive behavioural strategies or skills, and not to reinforce the problematic strategies, to "water the flowers, not the weeds". Mindfulness is drawn on heavily and skills are taught within the units of "distress tolerance", "emotion regulation" and "interpersonal effectiveness". DBT is an evidence-based treatment for emotionally unstable or borderline personality disorder (EUPD/BPD) and is included in the NICE Guideline for the treatment of BPD (National Institute for Clinical Excellence (NICE, 2009).

Cognitive Analytic Therapy

Cognitive Analytic Therapy (CAT) was developed by Anthony Ryle, a General Practitioner and Consultant Psychotherapist, in the late 1970s (Llewelyn, 2003). CAT examines the way a person thinks, feels, and acts, and the events and relationships that underlie these experiences (often from childhood or earlier in life). As its name suggests, it draws together ideas and understanding from different therapies and attachment theory. It mainly focuses on relationship patterns and is based on the idea that our early life experiences influence the way we relate to other people and how we treat ourselves. This means that sometimes patterns of behaviour, or our expectations of other people's behaviour, can develop into unhealthy or unhelpful repeating patterns, as well as those that are healthy and helpful. Diagrams or "maps" are developed that clarify both the problematic patterns and the healthy/helpful ones in order to start to develop new more helpful patterns and develop a better relationship with self and others.

Narrative and Solution Focussed Therapies

Narrative therapy was developed by Michael White and David Epston as a form of family therapy in 1989 (Besley, 2002). Narrative approaches emphasise that the *problem* is the problem, not the person, and focuses on the stories we tell about ourselves and others, and how these shape our reality. When narratives are problem-saturated, identities can become dominated by the problems. Narrative therapy seeks out knowledge and skills that run counter to the problem-saturated story which, with curiosity and exploration, can be richly described and developed. This allows people to not only find their voice but to use their voice for good, helping them to become experts in their own lives, and to live in a way that reflects their goals and values. Individuals feel more empowered to make changes in their thought patterns, behaviour, and "rewrite" their life story for a future that reflects who they really are, what they are capable of, and what their purpose is, separate from their problems.

Solution focussed therapy was developed by Steve de Shazer and Insoo Kim Berg in collaboration with their colleagues at the Milwaukee Brief Family Therapy Centre beginning in the late 1970s (Franklin et al., 2011). It is based upon social constructivist ideas and Wittgensteinian philosophy. Similarly to narrative therapy, it explores exceptions to the problem and builds upon individuals' strengths which they may have become disconnected from in the context of the problems. The approach incorporates positive psychology principles and practices, and the therapy is driven forward by a future vision and constructing solutions together rather than focusing on problems.

Systemic Therapies

Systemic therapy has its roots in the development of family therapies, which originated in the 1950s (Lorås et al., 2017). Systemic therapy focuses on interactions and relationships, examining the patterns that keep the problem going. The concept of systemic therapy springs from systems theory, which looks at how parts of a system affect one another to sustain the stability and equilibrium of the whole. Interactions are viewed as circular rather than linear in terms of cause and effect. The therapist's role is to introduce creative "nudges" to help systems change themselves. There are several different models contained within the systemic paradigm with a broad evolution of thinking from viewing the therapist as an expert external to the system (first order approaches based on cybernetics), to viewing the therapist as joining the system (second order approaches influenced by social constructivism), to a post-modern active process of meaning-making between therapist and other group members (third order approaches). Family interventions are a form of systemic psychotherapy, which are an evidence-based intervention for people who have experienced psychosis, (National Institute for Clinical Excellence, NICE, 2014) and for people with eating disorders (in particular youths with anorexia nervosa, Gorrell, 2019). Therapy interventions are designed to help clients become aware of their specific family "dance" and how they might change their steps.

Psychoeducation

Psychoeducation is an evidence-based therapeutically-informed intervention for service users and their loved ones that provides information and support to better understand and cope with illness. It can include teaching about the nature of mental illness including exacerbating factors such as poor sleep hygiene or substance misuse, developing problem-solving skills, building upon communication and assertiveness skills, making relapse-prevention plans and engaging in crisis management and suicide-prevention. Psychoeducation can be an important and necessary stage prior to psychotherapy which orientates the patient towards the need for therapy and builds motivation to engage. Unlike the previously described therapies, psychoeducation can be delivered by practitioners without training in a specific therapeutic modality.

What Makes a Therapy Effective?

Given the many different models of psychological therapy, one might reasonably wonder what makes a therapy effective? Much research has investigated the common factors of therapies and those that have the most significant positive impact (known as common factors models). Models vary, but some suggest that there are four key aspects of psychological therapies in terms of having a positive outcome (Sprenkle & Blow, 2004). These are proposed to be;

- The therapeutic relationship
- Client and extra-therapeutic factors
- Models and techniques
- Expectancy/hope.

It has been suggested that client and extra-therapeutic factors accounts for 40% of therapeutic change (Miller et al., 1997). This might include the personality of the service user, and other factors in their life. The therapeutic alliance is thought to account for around 30% of change (Miller et al., 1997). Therapeutic alliance is partly about the attachment between the therapist and the client; the genuine, warm, and supportive relationship that enables a therapeutic safe space to be created. It is also mediated by an agreement over the goals of therapy, and an agreement about the methods to achieve those goals (Bordin, 1979). The other two aspects, models/techniques, and expectancy/hope are thought to contribute about 15% each to change (Miller et al., 1997).

Other key considerations are readiness, ability, and willingness of the service user to engage in therapy. These are factors that could be assessed by the treating service, but it is helpful to have a broad understanding of the service user's motivation to engage and any factors that might need to be held in mind for the delivery of therapy such as literacy and cognitive ability. Factors such as literacy problems, learning difficulties, neurodiversity, and cognitive functioning are not necessarily barriers to psychological treatment, but could require the treating service to have the capacity to make adaptations to therapy delivery. Readiness and willingness are dynamic factors which can change over time and therefore should be revisited periodically. There is also evidence that mandated therapy can be effective, (Hachtel, Vogel & Huber, 2019), although this is not always the case and attendance does not necessarily equate with effective engagement.

It is our experience that patients detained in hospital who are acutely mentally unwell can value and make use of a therapeutic space prior to having identified goals or even prior to agreeing about the need for therapy. Often they are experiencing the world as frightening, chaotic, unpredictable, and overwhelming. Sometimes they want the opportunity to talk but can only tolerate a few minutes initially. Whilst obtaining consent for engagement in therapeutic work is essential, it also sometimes necessary to spend weeks, or even months, on the engagement process, actively building trust and rapport with the client by providing a regular reliable space and being empathetic and non-judgmental as they detail their experiences and tell their story. This phase of the work might include some psychoeducation, or might be predominantly listening, before reaching a point of agreeing goals for the therapy and the model of therapy.

What do we expect from a therapist to enable the best possible outcome for the service user? The training, experience, competence, and confidence of the therapist are factors which contribute to the sense of containment and purpose of the therapy. Maintenance of appropriate boundaries is crucial for the safety of the therapy and the therapeutic relationship. Striking a balance between the warmth, encouragement, and genuine positive regard to support the therapeutic relationship, with holding professional boundaries to ensure a safe experience for the service user, requires skill and experience. When a therapy becomes "stuck", it is often the case that something has gone awry with the therapeutic alliance. Ongoing supervision of the therapeutic work enables the therapist to reflect upon their own practice and make sense of any difficulties in the process or feelings evoked in themselves (which might be framed as transference and countertransference using a psychoanalytic model). It is important that therapists are registered with a regulatory body, to demonstrate up-to-date competence and to provide the service user with assurance about their practice. Regulatory bodies set out the "values and standards expected of any professional psychotherapist... they also give an indication to clients and patients of what they can expect from their therapists and, more importantly, what they can expect not to happen" (Adshead, 2010, p. 6).

Which Therapy?

It is important that a therapeutic intervention is evidence-based, in order to ensure that the service user is receiving an intervention that is likely to help and is unlikely to cause harm. However, evidencing therapeutic effectiveness is complicated in itself. The NICE guidelines attempt to do this work for us, by reviewing the evidence base for therapies and issuing guidance about which therapies are evidenced to be most effective for which areas of need. For instance, currently the NICE guidelines suggest CBT for psychosis or Family Intervention as the evidence-based interventions for people experiencing psychosis (National Institute for Clinical Excellence, NICE, 2022). In practice, the situation can be more nuanced, and new therapies are continually being developed to help with specific problems, and an evidence base may be being developed for some time before it reaches the NICE guidelines. It is also the case that in clinical practice sometimes an integrative approach is used, in which the clinician integrates aspects of different approaches when this best serves the service user and the formulation.

Perhaps it is most essential to consider the target or need for the therapeutic intervention, which is usually an emotional response or behaviour that is causing distress to self and/or others. The questions are then which interventions are recommended for this and what is available locally. When recommending a therapeutic intervention it is prudent to not be too specific or narrow in identifying a therapeutic approach, as this may not be easily available. If the focus is on the desired outcomes then the treating team can consider what resources available may meet the need.

Service user preference is also a relevant consideration. In the community, when accessed as a private client, the service user can be strongly influenced by their preference. They might consider whether they have a preference for group or individually delivered therapies, whether they wish to see their therapist online or in person, and they are free to seek a treatment model that resonates for them. In NHS services, and when being treated under section of the Mental Health Act, service users are likely to have more restricted choice. If they are being treated in hospital then they will have access to the psychological therapies available at that hospital. However, even within that more limited scope, they may still hold a preference within the options that are available to them.

It should also be noted that some service users do not want to engage in talking therapy but can still be successful in maintaining positive change through a combination of other factors such as external inhibitors to risk behaviours, medication compliance or establishing meaningful activities and improved social relations.

Offending/Risk

When individuals have caused harm to others, it may be recommended that they undertake psychological therapy with the aim of reducing their risk to others (for example, targeting violent or sexually harmful behaviours). This can be delivered in groups or individually. Much of this form of therapy is delivered in prisons and as such is often delivered in groups, both harnessing the power of group therapy and creating a cost-effective intervention. These offence focused groups usually draw on a range of models and approaches including psychoeducation, CBT, DBT, strengths-based approaches and compassionate-focused approaches. Evidence suggests that cognitive behavioural programmes that address dynamic criminogenic risk factors can be effective in reducing recidivism (Tomlinson, 2018). In UK prisons, much data is collected aiming to aid investigation of the evidence for the effectiveness of these interventions, and as such the interventions change reasonably regularly in order to maximise the effective aspects. For instance, the Core Sex Offender Treatment Programme (SOTP) was withdrawn (and replaced with an alternative intervention) following research that found that it either did not reduce sexual offending as it intended to, or that the true impact of the programme was not detected by the research (Mews et al., 2017).

It is a challenge of this kind of intervention that the individual may not always be motivated to engage in a therapy, for instance to change patterns of antisocial behaviour. It is an additional challenge that the therapist holds a dual role; not only are they attempting to hold the best interests of their client at the heart of their work, but they also have a responsibility to protect the public, and these two imperatives may not always go hand-in-hand. This tension is not always to the fore and for some service users there will be an alignment between their goals and reducing risk to others; that is interventions aimed helping people to live better lives, and not simply targeting isolated risk factors, will increase individuals' abilities to meet their own needs in a pro-social manner and decrease risk of offending (Barnao, Ward & Robertson, 2015).

It is beyond the scope of this chapter to go into detail about the application, effectiveness, and complexities, of psychotherapies aimed to reduce risk to others. However, the same principles apply in that the starting place is an assessment and formulation which makes sense of the presentation and identifies key targets for intervention.

Availability of Psychotherapies

Availability of psychotherapies varies enormously, dependent on numerous factors including setting/service, geography, staffing levels and vacancies, local structures, and budget for external providers. It will be likely to assist in the proposal of treatment pathways if availability of services are checked before recommendations are made for specific therapies.

Inpatient settings tend to have larger teams of psychologists and psychological therapists, as service users in inpatient settings are likely to have a higher level of need for therapeutic intervention to support their recovery and progress back to the community. The provision in community teams, whether specifically forensic teams or general adult mental health teams, usually lends itself to support via consultation and more limited availability for direct therapy.

Additionally, there may be junior or in-training staff members in the psychological therapies team whose level of training limits the type and scope of therapeutic interventions that they are able to offer. NHS organisations are responsible for clinical governance relating to patient care, including ensuring that practitioners have appropriate training and supervision for their role. NHS organisations are also responsible for service delivery.

Maximising Service User Engagement

In recent years there has been a powerful and important movement to maximise service user engagement and choice. It is important that therapeutic treatment plans are "done with, not done to", and that service users feel empowered, informed and respected to make choices. This is particularly important in mental health services and inpatient services, where often service users have historically felt disempowered, and current literature highlights the importance of building recovery capital to support personal recovery (Leamy et al., 2011).

One way in which organisations attend to this is by providing information about the therapies available, sometimes referred to as "menus of interventions", and information about consent to treatment. Written consent to engagement in therapy is the gold standard after receiving accessible information about the treatment. As outlined earlier, sometimes the engagement process with distressed inpatients can be protracted, and presence in the therapy room is initially regarded as consent to exploring the utility of talking therapy.

In group therapies, a powerful way of harnessing service user engagement is when those who have completed therapies return to the group as a "graduate" or "mentor". Substance use treatment is an area in which service user engagement is quite advanced, where much of the therapy for substance misuse being provided or at least supported by peers who have lived experience and have used services themselves. Perhaps the most well-known example of a peer-led group aimed at behavioural change is the 12-step programme for people recovering from addictions (e.g. Donovan, 2013).

Equality, Diversity and Inclusion (EDI)

It is clearly of paramount importance, and a responsibility on all clinicians, to ensure that their practice as a therapist is inclusive, acknowledges and respects diversity, and works towards expanding access. Cultural competence is an important concept in healthcare services. It can be described as aiming "to make health care services more accessible, acceptable and effective for people from diverse ethnocultural communities" (Kirmayer, 2012).

This can be a complex challenge. It is acknowledged that the population of psychologists in the UK are predominantly white, middle class and university educated, and also largely female. Data from 2023 indicates that registered psychologists are 84% white and 79% female (HCPC, 2023). The situation with subgroups such as Forensic Psychologists is even more extreme, with data showing that Forensic Psychologists are 87% white and 81% female (Bowes, 2023) and this is combined with the reverse situation in the client group, in that clients of forensic psychologists – those within the Criminal Justice System – are disproportionately likely to be BAME males. Clearly there is work to be done in improving access to the profession in order to provide a more diverse workforce; and in the meantime, it is clearly important for the predominantly white, university educated workforce to be mindful of their privilege and how this might impact their approach to their work.

Psychologists and psychotherapists will find themselves needing to offer their services to those for whom English is not their first language. It is important that people have equal access to services, and this is an interesting and important challenge for a talking therapy. If it is thought that the person would benefit from a talking therapy, or if it is their preference over other treatment options, then it is crucial that psychologists and therapists work to make their services accessible. The use of interpreters is one common option, which in itself raises some issues regarding the type of content the interpreter may be exposed to, and the level of training and supervision they receive to aid with processing the material, and also how the trio of service user, interpreter and therapist may address any risk of drift in cultural understanding through the process of interpreting.

Conclusion

In this chapter, we have aimed to summarise the (perhaps bewildering) range of psychological therapies potentially available and provide something of a roadmap for how to navigate the abundance of potential options. In doing so, we have considered the common factors that make therapies effective, and the importance of seeking evidence-based therapies with competent and registered therapists. We have summarised the importance of service user choice and engagement, and the importance of the therapeutic relationship between therapist and service user.

When considering pathways for psychological treatment, broadly the steps we have outlined are:

- Identify targets for intervention via assessment and formulation (which may already be in place or may need to be a recommendation)
- Identify what has already been tried and previous progress made
- Establish the necessity of making changes prior to discharge from hospital or supervision, and whether some targets for intervention can be safely left to patient choice
- Find out what psychological interventions are evidence-based for the target issues (considering available treatments and efficacy)
- Find out what is available in the local services that will be undertaking care and treatment
- Make recommendations for treatment with due consideration to above factors; and ensure to consider equality, diversity, and inclusion (EDI) issues and patient choice
- Avoid being too prescriptive and allow some leeway for treating teams to contribute to the decision-making process.

References

Adshead, G. (2010). Ethics and psychotherapy. In P. Fonagy (Ed.), *Digest of National Occupational Standards for Psychological Therapies.* Skills for Health.

Arntz, A., Jacob, G. A., Lee, C. W., Brand-de Wilde, O. M., Fassbinder, E., Harper, R. P., ... & Farrell, J. M. (2022). Effectiveness of predominantly group schema therapy and combined individual and group schema therapy for borderline personality disorder: A randomized clinical trial. *JAMA Psychiatry*, *79*(4), 287–299.

Barnao, M., Ward, T., & Robertson, P. (2015). The good lives model: A new paradigm for forensic mental health. *Psychiatry, Psychology and Law*, *23*(2), 288–301.

Bateman, A., & Fonagy, P. (2010). Mentalization based treatment for borderline personality disorder. *World Psychiatry*, *9*(1), 11–5.

Beck, J. S., & Fleming, S. (2021). A brief history of Aaron T. Beck, MD, and cognitive behavior therapy. *Clinical Psychology in Europe*, *3*(2), e6701. https://doi.org/10.32872/cpe.6701

Besley, A. C. (2002). Foucault and the turn to narrative therapy. *British Journal of Guidance and Counselling*, *30*(2), 125–143.

Bordin, E. S. (1979). The generalizability of the psychoanalytic concept of the working alliance. *Psychotherapy: Theory, Research & Practice, 16*(3), 252.

Bowes, N. (2023). Chair's Message. *Division of Forensic Psychology Newsletter*, August 2023.

Cook, S. C., Schwartz, A. C., & Kaslow, N. J. (2017). Evidence-based psychotherapy: Advantages and challenges. *Neurotherapeutics, 3*, 537–545.

de Klerk, N., Abma, T. A., Bamelis, L. L., & Arntz, A. (2017). Schema therapy for personality disorders: A qualitative study of patients' and therapists' perspectives. *Behavioural and Cognitive Psychotherapy, 45*(1), 31–45.

Donovan, D. M., Ingalsbe, M. H., Benbow, J., & Daley, D. C. (2013). 12-step interventions and mutual support programs for substance use disorders: An overview. *Social Work in Public Health, 28*(3–4), 313–332. https://doi.org/10.1080/19371918.2013.774663

Franklin, C., Trepper, T. S., McCollum, E. E., & Gingerich, W. J. (Eds.). (2011). *Solution-Focused Brief Therapy: A Handbook of Evidence-Based Practice*. Oxford Academic.

Gorrell, S., Loeb, K. L., & Le Grange, D. (2019). Family-based treatment of eating disorders: A narrative review. *The Psychiatric Clinics of North America, 42*(2), 193–204. https://doi.org/10.1016/j.psc.2019.01.004

Hachtel, H., Vogel, T., & Huber, C. G. (2019). Mandated treatment and its impact on therapeutic process and outcome factors. *Front Psychiatry*, 10, 219. doi: 10.3389/fpsyt.2019.00219

Hayes, S. C. (2004). Acceptance and commitment therapy, relational frame theory, and the third wave of behavioral and cognitive therapies. *Behavior Therapy, 35*(4), 639–665.

Hayes, S. C., & Hofmann, S. G. (2021). "Third-wave" cognitive and behavioral therapies and the emergence of a process-based approach to intervention in psychiatry. *World Psychiatry, 20*(3), 363–375. PMID: 34505370; PMCID: PMC8429332. https://doi.org/10.1002/wps.20884

HCPC. (2023). *Diversity Data: Practitioner Psychologists – July 2023*. www.hcpc-uk.org

Johnstone, L., Boyle, M., Cromby, J., Dillon, J., Harper, D., Kinderman, P., Longden, E., Pilgrim, D., & Read J. (2018). *The Power Threat Meaning Framework: Overview*. British Psychological Society.

Kirmayer, L. J. (2012). Rethinking cultural competence. *Transcultural Psychiatry, 49*(2), 149–164.

Leamy, M., Bird, V., Le Boutillier, C., Williams, J., & Slade, M. (2011). 'A conceptual framework for personal recovery in mental health: Systematic review and narrative synthesis'. *British Journal of Psychiatry, 199*(6), 445–452.

Levy, K. (2009). Psychodynamic and psychoanalytic psychotherapy. In Richard, D & Huprich, S. (Eds.), *Clinical Psychology: Assessment, Treatment, and Research* (Chapter 8, pp.179–211). Academic Press.

Lilienfeld, S. O. & Arkowitz, H. (2012, September 1). Are all psychotherapies created equal? *Scientific American*. www.scientificamerican.com/article/are-all-psychotherapies-created-equal/

Linehan, M. M. (1993). *Skills Training Manual for Treating Borderline Personality Disorder*. Guilford Press.

Llewelyn, S. (2003). Cognitive analytic therapy: Time and process. *Psychodynamic Practice, 9*(4), 501–520.

Lorås, L., Bertrando, P., & Ness, O. (2017). Researching systemic therapy history: In search of a definition. *Journal of Family Psychotherapy, 28*(2), 134–149.

Mews, A., Di Bella, L., & Purver, M. (2017). Impact evaluation of the prison-based core sex Offender Treatment Programme. *Ministry of Justice Analytical Series*. At www.gov.uk/government/publications ISBN 978-1-84099-783-5

Miller, S. D., Duncan, B. L., & Hubble, M. A. (1997). *Escape from Babel: Toward a Unifying Language for Psychotherapy Practice*. Norton.

National Institute for Clinical Excellence (NICE) Clinical Guideline. (2009). Borderline personality disorder: Recognition and management. *BMJ*, 228, b93

National Institute for Clinical Excellence (NICE) Clinical Guideline. (2014). *Psychosis and Schizophrenia in Adults: Treatment and Management*. CG178; pubmed.ncbi.nlm.nih.gov

National Institute for Clinical Excellence (NICE) Guideline. (2022). *Depression in Adults: Treatment and Management*. NG222; nice.org.uk

Norcross, J. C. (Ed.). (2011). *Psychotherapy Relationships That Work* (2nd ed.). Oxford University Press.

Norcross, J. C., & Lambert, M. J. (2018). Psychotherapy relationships that work III. *Psychotherapy*, *55*(4), 303.

Sprenkle, D., & Blow A. (2004). Common factors and our sacred models. *Journal of Marital and Family Therapy*, *30*, 113–129.

Swales, M. A. (2009). Dialectical behaviour therapy: Description, research and future directions. *International Journal of Behavioral Consultation and Therapy*, *5*(2), 164–177. https://doi.org/10.1037/h0100878

Tomlinson, M. F. (2018). A theoretical and empirical review of dialectical behavior therapy within forensic psychiatric and correctional settings worldwide. *International Journal of Forensic Mental Health*, *17*(1), 72–95.

Woods, J. (2014). Principles of forensic group therapy. In J. Woods, & A. Williams (Eds.), *Forensic Group Psychotherapy: The Portman Clinic Approach* (pp. 3–31). Karnac Books.

Yalom, I. D., & Leszcz, M. (2005). *The Theory and Practice of Group Psychotherapy* (5th ed.). Basic Books.

Young, J. E., Klosko, J. S., & Weishaar, M. E. (2003). *Schema Therapy: A Practitioner's Guide*. Guilford Press.

4 Occupational Therapy in Context of Mental Health Services

Philip Jones

Introduction

In practice, it is often the case to associate occupational therapists (OT) with discharge planning in the context of care packages. Indeed, OT practitioners are frequently at the forefront of the assessment processes which allow adjustments to accommodation that might, for example, allow patients to return home aided by specialist equipment. Often this might involve adjustments to the physical environment in the form of stair lifts, railings or changes to baths/showers which allow a service user easier access. Whilst by no means being a complete understanding of the role of an OT, this sense that an OT is thinking about adaptions that might give a person greater freedom is a useful place to begin. The Royal College of Occupational Therapists (RCOT) (2024) describe occupational therapy as:

> Occupational therapy helps you live your best life at home, at work – and everywhere else. It's about being able to do the things you want and have to do. That could mean helping you overcome challenges learning at school, going to work, playing sport or simply doing the dishes. Everything is focused on your wellbeing and your ability to participate in activities.
>
> (RCOT, 2024, p1)

Thane (2009), highlights that ever since the 1950's there has been a general move towards trying to look after people in the community where possible. Even the 1959 Mental Health Act expresses the desire for "mentally ill people to live, as far as possible, in the community". Thane acknowledges that resources were limited but the desire to facilitate a life outside of hospital is one which has been a consistent feature of policy. This has continued through the likes of Stein and Test (1980), through the assertive outreach model which was a key part of the National service framework, (1999). In policy terms, this has been superseded by New Horizons (2009), and "No health without mental health" (2011), The preamble of No health without mental health includes the phrase:

> We know many of the factors that help people to recover from mental health problems and live the lives they want to lead" which brings us full circle to the RCOT description discussing that "it's about being able to do the things you want and have to do.

So mental health policies have consistently discussed service users living good productive lives for the last 50 years or more. Urish (2020), provides an initial discussion of the way in which occupational therapy has become an important part of the discussion around assessment feeding into planning and delivering care. As Urish highlights this was initially focused on occupational

DOI: 10.4324/9781003635543-5

status but has evolved to include questions of self-care, and of course over time, assessment has grown in complexity and nuance. This has included a move from more functional assessments around physical capabilities to taking account of the psychological and emotional factors that might be more evident in the cases of mental health service users. Macrae (2019) discussed occupational health in context of the environment within which someone lives, their identity, and social and cultural context. The evolving understanding of mental health, including research around the impact of hospitalisation, and the importance of health and wellbeing within the context of communities has impacted mental health practice as a whole, and as is illustrated by Macrae's corresponding impact on occupational health practice.

Mental Disorder and Causality

There are a number of key factors/experiences associated with the onset of mental illness. Read et al. (2004) set out to update the evidence base and gather the variety of research that illustrate the many and various factors which contribute to the development of mental illness. Read et al. believe that there has been an overemphasis on biology and genetics within psychiatry. They present their book as a response and balance to the crude and biologically reductive approaches that have dominated psychiatry for too long (a point of view that has a growing constituency and captured effectively in the work of Filer, 2019). As such they present a variety of studies and have gathered evidence investigating the factors which contribute to the development of mental illness. Specifically, Read argues that mental health hospitals have always been filled with poor people. This point is developed in context of a wider discussion about structural inequalities by Pinfold et al. (2024) Across the world studies have concluded that there is a clear correlation between poverty and rates of mental illness (for example in the recent work of Gonzales et al., 2023 within a Spanish context). Read et al. (2004), moves on to discuss urbanicity and gathers together a variety of studies reflecting that not only is schizophrenia specifically related to living within an urban environment, but also relationship between the length of time the person has lived within an urban environment and the increased risk of becoming schizophrenic. Krabbendam et al. (2021) argue that given that 55% of the world's population now live in cities it is important to explore in more detail the relationship between the urban environment and mental health. They offer an in-depth and multidisciplinary analysis of this phenomenon. Read also highlights the gross cultural incompetence evident within psychiatry around issues of culture. People from an ethnic minority are consistently shown to be far more likely to be diagnosed with a mental illness, again specifically schizophrenia than a native population. Ethnicity was found to be an even greater factor in determining outcomes of diagnosis for schizophrenia than socio-economic status. This is discussed by Filer (2019) in context of his experience but also drawing on statistics about migrants in a variety of other contexts e.g. Greenlanders in Denmark. Rosenberg (2015) highlights a variety of inequalities related to ethnicity in America that goes well beyond diagnosis of schizophrenia. Rosenberg asks the more pointed question as to whether this is cultural incompetence or just racism? Read et al. (2004), suggests that the only viable explanation for the massively disproportionate numbers of people from ethnic minority groups (mis)diagnosed with schizophrenia is quite simply cultural incompetence on behalf of a profession who in attempts to be systematic and objective fail to understand the subjective experiences of the people they are treating. Read et al. (2004), reflect the causal role of sexual abuse in a variety of mental illnesses. Read et al. argue that it has often been assumed that childhood sexual abuse is more associated with less severe psychiatric symptomology and less so with schizophrenia. They do not believe this to be true and draw together data from a variety of studies illustrating clear causal links between various forms of severe abuse, loss, and trauma and the development of psychosis. Werbeloff et al. (2021) support these findings and highlight the range of negative consequences in terms of mental health that stem from childhood sexual abuse including a range of symptoms and negative social experiences. Reed et al. argue that specifically child sexual abuse is associated with earlier first admissions and more lengthy admissions to psychiatric hospitals, with these people spending longer in seclusion, receiving more medication and being more likely to self-mutilate. Overall childhood sexual abuse is associated with more severe symptoms that are also more resistant to treatment (in the form of medication).

As such there is a very clearly researched and understood link between social context and the aetiology of mental illness. What is more Tyrer (2019) suggests that most chronic conditions (including mental health conditions) are sustained because they are associated with toxic circumstances. So as an example, someone who has been brought up in a very dysfunctional context might be better able to sustain a sense of positive wellbeing if they were not still living in a toxic setting (whether that be the original context or a similar replica resulting from repetitive life choices and behaviours). Tyrer acknowledges that the evidence for environmental interventions remains limited although the recent increase in use of social prescribing is an example where busy healthcare practitioners can be supported by often quite low-cost interventions.

Practical Intervention

The importance to occupational health is that the focus on very practical interventions is essential to good mental health practice. Macrae (2019), for example highlights that in adults aged 35–44 are some of the unhappiest in society due to money worries, work hassles, and loneliness. Typically, mental health service users are less likely to be working, and therefore, more likely to present with such concerns. Eklund et al. (2024), whilst agreeing with Tyrer (2019) that lots of interventions remain largely unevaluated, suggests that the best evidence focuses on lifestyle and occupation focused interventions. Eklund et al. (2024), provide several practical examples of evidence-based OT interventions in this regard which include supported employment and social recovery therapy which includes a focus on identifying meaningful activity. Atler and Fox (2021), highlight the way in which occupational therapy fits with the recovery model regarding bringing a focus on hope, identity, and purpose. Importantly, Atler and Fox highlight that interventions do not necessarily need to lead to full time employment and that research suggests that sometimes very ordinary activities can instil a sense of purpose, hope, and a more positive expression of self. Stemming from extensive experience in practice, I have often taken the view that routine and structure can be as effective as any more formal intervention. So many mental health colleagues would recognise the description of the service user who seems to have far too much time to think about things, and if for no other reason, needs activity to distract them from their own thoughts or to provide them with a useful avenue to direct their energies. Kirsch et al. (2019), has carried out a literature review to try and tackle the issue of needing evidence-based interventions. Kirsch et al. grouped together the key interventions for which they have been able to find clear evidence. Firstly, supported employment which focuses on reintegrating service users within employment. Similarly, supported education focuses mostly on post-secondary education and involved approaches such as peer mentoring. Kirsch et al. also recognise the importance of a variety of approaches to employment to support integration into the workplace. Secondly, there are a variety of psychoeducational approaches identified which have an evidence base and these include techniques to increase the capacity of the service users to manage themselves and develop routines that would aid moving toward employment. Finally, there are a variety of approaches grouped under the theme of creative occupations and activity. This is about involving service users in activities that begin to create a greater sense of structure, and the basic skills required within employment such as relationship building.

Having established what occupational therapy is and the kinds of evidence-based interventions that are recognised within the literature, we can begin to explore how these kinds of interventions can fit within the tribunal process. There is an expectation that if writing an in-patient nursing report the current nursing plan would be included, and this might include OT interventions. However, the social circumstances report needs to include the opportunities for employment and the support available for the patient if they were to be discharged from hospital. As the patient is currently subject to a section of the mental health act, the report will need to include some discussion around the service users history of employment, discussing any recent employment, and as a result of discussions with the service user reflect the expectations regarding employment. It is also worth returning to the work of Read et al. (2004), who remind us that a typical service user is more likely to be poorer, less well educated, and have a less well-developed social network. Filer (2019) illustrates this point throughout his book but specifically highlights the psychiatric system can be one which too frequently disempowers those within it. Beresford (2010) similarly discusses issues of stigma and provides examples of the way in which service users might be disempowered. I want to return us to the idea of "living your best life" from within our initial discussion of occupational therapy's purpose. Cummins (2018), highlights the way in which there is a social gradient in the extent of mental health problems. Many are unable to work (especially if in hospital) and if they can return to work then they face issues of discrimination. As such, it is unwise to simply suggest that the solution to most mental health service users struggles is for a return to work. Indeed, this insight is not new it is one of a number of key points made within the Marmott review, (2010). The impact of austerity made many of the factors that Marmott and others agree contribute to mental health problems even more prevalent. The pressure of living in poverty, debt, and in precarious accommodation contribute to the likelihood that someone will develop a mental health problem.

Anyone who has worked in mental health services will have stories to tell regarding the experiences of their service users, for example when regarding the relatively new work capabilities assessments. The idea behind this is that rather than simply discounting so many people from the workplace a much smaller proportion being unable to work meant that the state could reduce the commitments of the welfare state. Cummins (2018) argues that this was as much a political project as an economic one, and mental health service users were some of those most impacted. Cummins highlights that the work capability assessment has been linked to 590 suicides, over a quarter of a million self-reported mental health problems and nearly three quarters of a million additional prescriptions for anti-depressants. Obviously within the working age population there is need for interventions around employment but also around resilience, housing, and the management of finances. Given the cuts in services such as the citizens advice bureau it is really important to understand whether a service user is receiving appropriate support.

Direct Work

As nurses we discuss our role as advocate frequently but in my experience, this is often thought of mostly in context of clinical review processes and ensuring the voice of the patient is heard in multi-disciplinary team meetings, etc. This is clearly an important act of advocacy but given the loss of community support available and the strain on remaining services it is more likely than ever that some of our service users are not receiving support to which they are entitled. As such, the following is a rough guide to the kinds of things that might be expected within an in-patient setting and can be reported on:

1. **Assessment and Evaluation**: OTs conduct comprehensive assessments to understand patients' strengths, challenges, and functional abilities. This includes evaluating their daily living skills, social interactions, and emotional well-being. . A commonly used example is the recovery star which is widely used and Dickens et al. (2012) discuss this regarding the recovery model and validating tools measuring recovery.
2. **Goal Setting**: Collaboratively setting personalized, achievable goals that focus on enhancing patients' daily functioning and quality of life. Goals may include improving self-care skills, managing stress, or enhancing social participation. The nature of the in-patient setting will vary but there should be an expectation that staff having assessed the service users' needs are planning care appropriate in a person-centred manner. This might include something as simple as establishing a positive sleep routine and engagement with mealtimes in the early stages.
3. **Therapeutic Activities**: Utilizing meaningful activities (occupations) to promote engagement and skill development. This may include art therapy, group activities, or life skills training, helping patients express themselves and develop coping strategies. Again, this will depend on what is available within the context of the in-patient environment. One of the important aspects of the tribunal is that they need to make an assessment as to whether the current environment is suitable for the service user. It may be that the particular ward is largely focused on acute interventions, and the service user is at a point where they need opportunities to engage more consistently with meaningful activities. A tribunal does not only decide whether or not ongoing detention under a section of the Mental Health Act is necessary, but they can also make recommendations regarding referrals to more suitable environments if appropriate activities are not available. The author/presenter of the social report is tasked with providing sufficient information to the panel so that they can understand both the context in which the service user is detained and the activities that are available within that context.
4. **Coping Strategies**: Teaching patients effective coping mechanisms and stress management techniques to manage challenges related to their mental health conditions. This can include mindfulness practices, relaxation techniques, and problem-solving skills. This might be provided by specialist staff such as psychologists or could be provided by staff working on the ward. Whilst there is a need for appropriately trained and skilled practitioners, there are also activities that can be conducted by any staff on the ward. The author of the social report's task is to establish both what is available formally but also what might be provided at a more basic level through general discussion, 1:1's, and more informal group work.
5. **Social Skills Training**: Facilitating group sessions that promote social interaction and communication skills, helping patients build relationships and a support network within the hospital setting. As with the above encouraging interaction between service users, informal group activities and peer support is all part of life within a good in-patient ward. It may be that there is access to something like a basketball court or a small garden where small groups of service users can be encouraged to interact with one another, develop empathy, and relate to one another in the ways that they will need to within the wider community. It is the task of all staff to promote a sense of self awareness in their service users thus enabling them to be more aware of the feelings and wellbeing of those around them. Often within ward environments specific service users might assume particular roles in regard to others, and if there are ward meetings, then it might be that the other service users select a

representative to represent their views. This can be a positive opportunity to develop key skills that are transferable to many workplaces. Equally it might just be that staff encourage service users to be more aware of their appearance and to take a greater degree of pride in themselves.

6. **Discharge Planning**: Preparing patients for successful reintegration into their communities by developing discharge plans that include referrals to community resources, follow-up services, and continued support. One of the biggest challenges that can exist around discharge is establishing a clear plan that is beyond the boundaries of the ward environment, this requires collaboration with community teams and services that might not be available until discharged The transition needs to be carefully managed, and it is important to identify what support exists and how this can be initiated at the right time so that the service user can access the support they need from day one. The author of the report might consider what support is available outside the hospital and will need to assess whether sufficient engagement is evident. Services can appear inflexible, and the tribunal need to understand the very real issues that might be evident around discharge planning but also the efforts that are being made to overcome such issues.

7. **Family Involvement**: Engaging family members in the therapeutic process to enhance support systems, educate them about mental health conditions, and improve family dynamics. One of the big differences between working in the community and a hospital is that in the community if family are actively involved with the service user then whatever the relationship there is a strong likelihood that there is some form of contact. In the hospital it is often much more difficult to assess the service users support networks. A key part of the social report is to speak with the nearest relative, and this in itself will often provide insight into some of the family dynamics but over the past 25 years there has been a clear sense that healthcare requires not just treatment of the service user but support for carers and attention to the context in which they live (Tyrer, 2019). Informal carers are a vital resource and part of the tribunal process is showing recognition of their vital role. How are they being supported? What arrangements are made for staying connected with them? Are they invited to key meetings?

8. **Environmental Modifications**: Assessing and recommending changes to the physical and social environment to enhance patients' engagement and safety, both in the hospital and at home. Having spent many years working in the community there is a clear understanding that landlords, shopkeepers, barbers/hairdressers, and a whole raft of other local people play an important part in the lives of the service users we work with. Equally, the locality in which someone lives can be of real importance. Putting a service user back into the community where their only friends are drug users after they have got themselves off illicit substances is an obvious example of the need for services to work closely with housing providers to look at appropriate accommodation options. Issues of security and safety are important for anyone feeling vulnerable and returning to the community after a substantial period in hospital.

9. **Advocacy**: Advocating for patients' rights and needs within the healthcare system, ensuring they receive comprehensive and holistic care. Changes in legislation in recent years mean that advocacy has been a growth area and ensuring that service users have legal representation is of key importance but equally organisations like MIND and RETHINK provide advocacy to mental health service users. What efforts have been made to provide independent support to the service user?

10. **Interdisciplinary Collaboration**: Working closely with other healthcare professionals (psychologists, psychiatrists, nurses) to provide integrated care that addresses the

multifaceted nature of mental health. Engagement is complex as on occasions a service user might attend all of their appointments but say little about how things are going. Equally, due to lifestyle or wider circumstances, it can be that a service user is well intentioned but the chaos surrounding them makes getting to appointments regularly a challenge. What is important is that the author of a report explores thoroughly not just whether a service user attends their one to one's regularly on the ward but explores beyond this the apparent willingness to work with a variety of professionals.

Through these aspects, occupational therapy helps patients in in-patient mental health settings regain autonomy, improve their functioning, and enhance their overall well-being.

OT in Practice

The final section is going to provide a couple of examples based around two short case studies to demonstrate application of some of the discussion above into practice. In my career as an assertive outreach nurse, two of the most common types of service user were young service users (18–25) possibly having been referred after several years of treatment with an early intervention service. These service users were often quite unwell and due to having become unwell quite young they were often emotionally and socially quite immature sometimes leading to difficulties in their interactions with wider society. The biggest single challenge was finding them opportunities to engage with education and/or training to provide them with some structure and routine and the opportunity to compensate for the time spent in hospital (or even prison) and/or time spent being unwell living in the community. The second type of service user is older (40–60) and has already spent around half of their lives unwell and have been in and out of hospital.

The first example is a reasonably young man who had a diagnosis which included psychosis and substance misuse. During his teenage years, despite early signs of mental illness, he had become a very good sportsman and although he didn't do well academically at school, he had completed his education until 16. As his mental health symptoms had worsened during his late teenage years, he had become more withdrawn from his peers, and then probably as an attempt at self-medication he had started to use cannabis. This had resulted in a sharp escalation in his symptoms, coming to the attention of the local home treatment team, being the subject of debates about whether his symptoms were the result of cannabis or an underlying mental health problem, and eventually after several in-patient admissions, he was referred to the assertive outreach team. Since his first hospital admission (followed by regular admissions over the following years) he had not regularly played any sport and had largely succumbed to a life of minimal routine and considerable substance misuse. His symptoms were largely uncontrolled within the community due to his cannabis use, and as such his care team had sought funding for a period of locked door rehabilitation. His tribunals are frequently dominated by debates about diagnosis, his often challenging and somewhat antisocial behaviours, and risks associated with his discharge. The fact that he had no immediate accommodation available and his family although still involved don't know what to do to help him and are exhausted, means they don't feel able to offer any further support within the community. I should note that in this kind of scenario there is a likelihood that much of the discussion within the tribunal is likely to be focused on the risk of discharge The question of how he might ever succeed in living his best life, (RCOT, 2024), can seem a rather obtuse question. I would like to suggest that in this context the kinds of interventions discussed above can be an essential source of hope. At one stage this was clearly a sociable young man who enjoyed playing sport and was quite good at it, and rather than this being another example of the life that could have been, it can provide the basis for a whole raft of activity and positive motivation. Are their local clubs that he could be encouraged to engage with? Is it possible that by offering some incentives around the community and leave to do things that are a source of motivation these might be the basis for establishing a routine of activities that might be of interest? Writing a report for a young man such as this I would be interested in seeing whether a good initial assessment has been completed with a positive focus on strengths as well as the more obvious areas of challenge. How have these strengths/interests been incorporated into the care plan? Have the ward put in place a routine and structure involving practical activities built around the development of important routines including basic things such as making their bed and cleaning their room. Are there opportunities to learn how to cook in context of the ward and if so are they being supported to learn how to cook food that is culturally appropriate or at least food that they are likely to want to eat given the choice? What has been explored in terms of accommodation, what are the service users aspirations and is there a clear plan in place to get from the current circumstances to a point where independent living is viable?

The second person I want to talk about is a little older, sometimes has been married or remains so. There are often difficulties within the relationships that exist sometimes because of the mental health issues, and some that may have contributed to the development of the mental health issues. given that they are currently in hospital it might be presumed that there has been a pattern of regular admissions going back to their 20's or even earlier. Given the regular admissions (sometimes even when concordant with treatment) they will often be considered treatment resistant. In most cases even if they have wanted to do so there has been limited opportunity to work. Service users who have been employed have become unwell may have lost their jobs or they may never have worked.. The first question to explore is whether a detailed assessment has taken place exploring relationships and family life, employment history and the service user's aspirations. In my experience there are often issues with confidence and whilst there doesn't need to be in depth psychological input, there does need to be carefully-developed smart goals around social skills and coping strategies. If appropriate, family therapy might be offered to explore how the relationships between the service user and partner or wider family might be improved and made more constructive. De Witt (2014), notes that one of the identified domains of occupational therapy is making constructive use of free time. It may be the service user is close to retirement and has little interest in formal employment but there is still a need to carefully think about how they will spend their time on discharge. It might be that staff have some clear objectives, but the service user isn't yet well enough to engage, or it might be that staff are seeking to work with the service user to identify how they will fill their time on discharge. The important issue is that within your report you can capture a clear sense that these issues are being addressed. .

The Benefits of OT Practice

These cases represent two hugely different service users of different ages, genders, and whilst one might still be lacking in basic life skills to live independently, the other may have kept her home neat and tidy and had jobs in the past. Guerrero et al. (2024) discuss some of the key contributions to discussions of what constitutes recovery in context of mental health through drawing on systematic reviews and their own engagement with experts by experience. They highlight the way in which recovery can be captured in at least two distinct ways – clinical recovery and personal recovery. Clinical recovery focuses on emerging from professionally led services whilst personal recovery focuses on self-determination and a combination of reduced symptoms and a return to a positive level of functioning. There is a very real sense that in terms of each of the case studies above both of these aspects can be understood in context of engagement with OT activities alongside the work of the wider MDT. Building positive relationships outside of services whether through social groups or work activities creates an opportunity to re-engage with parts of society that mental health service users often withdrawer from (or are withdrawn from). The development of basic social skills and the opportunity to practice them within the community is a process of re-establishing the persons place within society as a full member of it. The symptoms of mental illness often led to rejection or withdrawal from society in some form and the role of OT here can be seen as one of facilitating a journey of re-establishing that sense of full personhood and full membership of society. The negative cycle of increasing symptoms, dislocation and disconnection which so often creates a downward spiral is reversed by purposeful engagement with the community, meaningful connections with other human beings and a very practical improvement in symptoms stemming from purposeful activity. Alongside the other parts of the MDT it should be the ultimate goal of OT to contribute to this positive vision of recovery.

Conclusion

I hope already that you have made connections between the definition of occupational therapy discussed earlier and how this might relate to each of these people. In both cases assessment needs to be genuinely bio-psychosocial going well beyond issues of diagnosis and medical/psychological treatment. Care planning should be person centred and reflective of strengths as well as needs, with a focus on recovery and a pathway towards a purposeful life within the community. Most importantly the care planning should recognise the person's potential to live a full life within the community and there should be evidence that this is the goal. What this constitutes will look different for each service user, but your task is to offer a neutral analysis of the extent to which this is evident. Psychiatric services are very capable of getting caught up with the immediate issues of medication concordance or management of symptoms and whilst there is nothing wrong with this as a primary focus in the early stages of detention the tribunal process demands that consideration is given to what happens next. Your report is an opportunity to ensure that care is holistic, and planning involves a future beyond hospital which is so important for instilling hope into service users who might be frustrated and distressed at their present circumstances.

References

Agius, M., and Agius, M., 2021. Traumatic events, sexual abuse and mental illness. *Psychiatria Danubina*, 33, pp. S19–S26.

Atler, K.E., and Fox, A.L., 2021. Mental health consumers' perspectives on using an occupation-focused assessment to initiate change in everyday activities. *British Journal of Occupational Therapy*, 84(8), pp. 497–506.

Beresford, P., 2010. *A straight talking introduction to being a mental health service user.* Monmouth: PCCS.

Cummins, I., 2018. The Impact of austerity on mental health service provision: a UK perspective. *International Journal of Environmental Research Public Health*, 15, p. 15.

De Witt, P., 2014. Creative ability: a model for individual and group occupational therapy for clients with psychosocial dysfunction. In Crouch, R., Alers, V., eds. *Occupational therapy in psychiatry and mental health.* Chichester: John Wiley.

Dickens, G., Weleminsky, J., Onifade, Y., and Sugarman, P., 2012. Recovery Star: validating user recovery. *The Psychiatrist*, 36(2), pp. 45–50.

Eklund, M., Parsonage-Harrison, J., and Argentzell, E., 2024. Occupation- and lifestyle-based mental health interventions – a hallmark for the occupational therapy profession? *British Journal of Occupational Therapy*, 87(7), pp. 395–397.

Filer, N., 2019. *This book will change your mind about mental health – a journey into the heartland of psychiatry.* London: Faber & Faber.

González, L., et al., 2023. Poverty, social exclusion, and mental health: the role of the family context in children aged 7–11 years INMA mother-and-child cohort study. *European Child & Adolescent Psychiatry*, 32(2), pp. 235–248.

Guerrero, E., M. Barrios, H. M. Sampietro, A. Aza, J. GÓMEZ-Benito, and G. Guilera. 2024. Let's talk about recovery in mental health: An International Delphi study of experts by experience. *Epidemiology and Psychiatric Sciences* **33,** e41. https://doi.org/10.1017/S2045796024000490.

Hemphill, B.J., Urish, C. eds, 2020. *Assessments in occupational therapy mental health: an integrative approach.* 4th ed. Thorofare, NJ: SLACK Incorporated.

Kirsh, B., et al., 2019. Occupational therapy interventions in mental health: a literature review in search of evidence. *Occupational Therapy in Mental Health*, 35(2), pp. 109–156.

Krabbendam, L., et al., 2021. Understanding urbanicity: how interdisciplinary methods help to unravel the effects of the city on mental health. *Psychological Medicine*, 51(7), pp. 1099–1110.

MacRae, A., 2019. *Cara and MacRae's psychosocial occupational therapy: an evolving practice.* 4th ed. New York: Routledge.

Marmot, M.F., 2010. *Society, healthy lives, the Marmot review*. London: Department of Health. Available at: www.parliament.uk/documents/fair-society-healthy-lives-full-report.pdf [accessed on 18 October 2024]

New horizons – a shared vision for mental health, 2009. (online). Available at: https://data.parliament.uk/DepositedPapers/Files/DEP2009-3023/DEP2009-3023.pdf [accessed 08 October 2024]

No Health Without Mental Health, 2011. A cross-government mental health outcomes strategy for people of all ages (online). Available at: https://assets.publishing.service.gov.uk/media/5a7c348ae5274a25a914129d/dh_124058.pdf [accessed 08 October 2024]

Pinfold, V., et al., 2024. Public perspectives on inequality and mental health: a peer research study. *Health Expectations: An International Journal of Public Participation in Health Care and Health Policy*, 27(1). pp. 1–15

Read, J., Mosher, L.R., and Benthall, R.P. eds, 2004. *Models of madness.* London and New York: Routledge.

Romans, S.E., Martin, J.L., Anderson, J.C., Herbison, G.P., and Mullen, P.E., 1995. Sexual abuse in childhood and deliberate self harm. *American Journal of Psychiatry*, 152(9), pp. 1336–1342.

Rosenberg, L., 2015. Is the problem cultural incompetence or racism? *The Journal of Behavioral Health Services & Research*, 42(4), pp. 414–416. doi: 10.1007/s11414-015-9481-8. PMID: 26354367

Royal College of Occupational Therapy, 2024. *What is occupational therapy?* (online). Available at: www.rcot.co.uk/about-occupational-therapy/what-is-occupational-therapy [accessed 08 June 2024]

Stein, L.I., and Test, M.A., 1980. Alternative to mental hospital treatment. I. Conceptual model, treatment program and clinical evaluation. *Archives of Psychiatry*, 37, pp. 392–397.

Thane, P., 2009. Memorandum submitted to the house of commons' health committee inquiry: Social care (online). Available at: www.historyandpolicy.org/docs/thane_social_care.pdf [accessed 08 October 2024]

The National Service Framework for Mental Health, 1999. Quality Standard for Menatl Health Services (online). Available at: https://assets.publishing.service.gov.uk/media/5a7a050040f0b66eab99926f/National_Service_Framework_for_Mental_Health.pdf [accessed 08 October 2024]

Tyrer, P., 2019. Nidotherapy: a cost-effective systematic environmental intervention. *World Psychiatry*, 18(2), 144–145. PMID: 31059613; PMCID: PMC6502418. doi: 10.1002/wps.20622

Werbeloff, N., et al., 2021. Childhood sexual abuse in patients with severe mental illness: demographic, clinical and functional correlates. *Acta Psychiatrica Scandinavica*, 143(6), pp. 495–502.

5 Nursing Care and Support

Helen Rees, Victoria Tracey and Catherine Stobbs

Introduction

Registered mental health nurses, and learning disability nurses, make up a significant proportion of the mental healthcare workforce (Gilburt and Mallorie, 2024). They also work across the lifespan and in a variety of settings, often providing care over a full 24-hour period. Since nurses are generally considered to be the closest healthcare workers to patients, both in terms of physical proximity and time spent together, they frequently take a leading role in assessing, delivering, and coordinating mental and physical healthcare. Being so integrated in patient care, however, makes it difficult to measure the importance of mental health nurses and makes defining their role particularly difficult (Hurley et al., 2022). What seems to set mental health nursing apart from other disciplines is the ability to provide care according to a patient-centred, bio-psycho-social-spiritual model of mental distress and, revise and implement care plans (developed following a model of coproduction) according to patient need. However, often the most visible aspects of the mental health nursing role are safety critical elements e.g. carrying out therapeutic observations, which are more likely to involve coercive practice and/or enforcing restrictions. Therefore, this chapter will explore the application of mental health nursing by providing an overview of relevant interventions and the role of nurses in upholding the principles of the Mental Health Act 1983 (amended 2007). It is also aligned to the standards by the nursing regulatory body framework which outlines the skill and knowledge expected from mental health nurses when working with others to plan and deliver evidence-based interventions.

Nursing and Psychological Therapies

Providing psychological interventions is a core part of the mental health nursing role and can take several forms for example, brief interventions, administering psychological therapies as an extended role (or under supervision) or co-facilitating interventions with colleagues. To achieve this, all registered nurses are expected to be skilled at so-called "active listening". Active listening supports emotional containment and has an important function in de-escalation, distress tolerance, and risk reduction (Cutler et al., 2020; NICE, 2015). The NHS England Inpatient Culture of Care Standards (2024) also recognise the importance of active listening in promoting hope and recovery. These sessions are not restricted to formal listening activities and should be patient-led, wherever possible. Patients receiving mental health treatment in the community also benefit from active listening and a 1:1 session with nurses. Nurses in assertive outreach teams, for example, work predominantly with patients who have experienced barriers accessing treatment and may use a 1:1 session to provide care in a more accessible and patient-centred manner e.g. by supporting patients to access social and leisure activities (Veitch, Strong and

DOI: 10.4324/9781003635543-6

Armstrong, 2017). Active listening is therefore one of the cornerstones of positive therapeutic relationships. Developing positive therapeutic relationships with patients also requires nurses to demonstrate unconditional positive regard and respect for the patient's agency and their own expertise. By developing trust and working collaboratively, mental health nurses can gain more information about their patients' strengths, coping skills, and vulnerabilities, which ultimately allows them to create more accurate risk assessments and formulations and, as a result, provide higher quality care.

In 2018, the Nursing and Midwifery Council (NMC) revised the standards of nursing proficiency in the Future Nurse Standards (NMC, 2018). Annexe A, of this document outlines the communication and relationship management skills all registered nurses are expected to possess. These include motivational interviewing, solution focused therapy, reminiscence therapy, talking therapies, de-escalation strategies and techniques, cognitive behavioural therapy techniques, play therapy, distraction and diversion techniques, and positive behaviour support.

Motivational interviewing was initially developed by substance misuse services to facilitate positive behavioural change and reduce the risks associated with alcohol consumption/ recreational drug use (Miller, 2023). It is an intervention that uses open questioning, strengths recognition, reflection, and summarising to explore motivation to change, actions needed to act on this motivation and the strengths a person has to take action (Miller and Rollnick, 2013). In addition to its original use, motivational interviewing has also been shown to be effective at promoting various other health behaviours including smoking cessation and medication adherence. By recognising that internal motivation is key to behavioural change, motivational interviewing is less likely to be perceived by patients as nagging or judgmental.

Solution focused therapy may be suitable for patients who feel frustrated/disillusioned by the focus given to their symptoms and/or things they have been unable to achieve (Proudlock and Sanghvi, 2017). It does this by setting clear, achievable, and realistic goals based on the patient's strengths (Jerome et al., 2023). By focussing on an individual's strengths, resources and non-problem talk, solution focused therapy can support people experiencing mental distress by rebuilding their self-esteem and sense of health autonomy.

Cognitive behavioural therapy (commonly referred to as CBT) works by exploring the links between an individual's thoughts, feelings, and behaviour (Allen, 2020). By understanding these areas better (and how they interact), it may be possible to formulate interventions which reduce an individual's distress (Lopez et al., 2019). This can be particularly helpful for mental distress generated by cyclical patterns of unhelpful thought/behaviour which reinforce each other. Even nurses without formal CBT training should be able to identify common thinking errors as well as biases and work with patients to challenge these when they are causing distress, (Better health, every mind matters, NHS, n.d.).

In addition to the structured psychological interventions described above, nurses should be able to promote short-term and long-term distress tolerance using fewer formal techniques. Short-term distress management, for example, may involve temporarily increasing the restrictions placed on a patient e.g., their level of nursing observations, managing the environment by removing risky objects/conducting room searches, or the use of seclusion. Patients who are experiencing distress secondary to intrusive or ruminating thoughts may also benefit from interventions that involve distraction techniques; effective and long-term distraction plans should be coproduced with patients and based on their individual needs. These might include guided relaxation (to distract from anxious ruminations), sensory boxes (to distract from thoughts about self-harm), or writing affirmation cards (to distract from persecutory hallucinations or anorexic thoughts).

De-escalation is an essential nursing skill that may include elements of distraction and redirection (Hallett and Dickens, 2015). To be successful, nurses need to engage in dynamic risk assessments and be familiar with an individual's early indicators of violence and aggression. Short term de-escalation strategies may include reducing environmental stimuli, mediating tone, and content of speech and meeting patient needs (NICE, 2015). Managing longer term risks should also include identifying contributory factors to historical aggression and violence, evaluating de-escalation techniques used previously, and supporting patients at risk of aggression and violence to access CBT or anger management programmes, (NICE, 2015). It is important to note that some people experience mental health services as restrictive, coercive, and stressful meaning that the presence of mental health staff and the mental health environment itself may elevate risk. It is therefore important that nursing documentation is clear about possible causal factors of violence and aggression and that steps are taken to reduce their impact where practicable.

Psychoeducation supports patients to understand their mental health challenges and their impact. This can be achieved by explaining the stress-vulnerability model of mental illness (Zubin and Spring, 1977) and/or the concept of a "stress bucket" (Mental Health UK, 2018). These models suggest that mental illnesses develop as a result of the interaction between vulnerabilities an individual may have (for example, a strong family history of mental illness), and stressors they are exposed to (such as bereavement or abuse). By using this approach, recovery work typically focuses on acknowledging vulnerability, reducing stressors and increasing resilience, (Brennan, 2023), for example, creating a timeline of significant events that preceded the individual becoming unwell and achieving recovery, (Marland et al., 2011). Timelines help patients by identifying significant stressors/resilience building activities and their so-called "early warning signs". It is generally accepted that most people have a period of time before a relapse where they demonstrate signs that they may becoming unwell. These signs (which occur before an episode of mental distress) are person-specific and generally subtler than the symptoms observed when some is acutely unwell. Examples include poor sleep, social withdrawal, and concentration difficulties. Training patients and their carers to recognise early warning signs allows them to seek appropriate support at an earlier stage, and is associated with better health outcomes, (Birchwood, Spencer and McGovern, 2000). This commonly involves the co-production of a relapse prevention and staying well plan, in which the patient agrees what steps should be taken to reduce their stressors/increase their resilience (in the event that their mental health deteriorates) to reduce the risk of them requiring more intensive or restrictive treatment e.g. hospital admission.

Formal observation underpins the nursing contribution to formal reports and assessments and includes monitoring the location and mental state of patients receiving care in inpatient settings. This can range from checking on a patient hourly, to ensuring that several members of staff are within arm's reach of a patient at all times (including during bathroom use). Whilst the level of observation required is typically determined by the multidisciplinary team (according to perceived risk), it is usually the nursing team who are responsible for ensuring that formal observations are conducted and documented according to organisational policy. Since there are no universally-agreed naming conventions for the different levels of observation, it is also essential that nurses clarify this information when working in new or unfamiliar environments. It should also be clear in any report what level of observation is a person is under. Patients may find observations less restrictive if nursing staff offer meaningful engagement during observation periods. This may include engaging in some of the psychological interventions discussed earlier in this chapter or informal activities such as watching films, accessing outside spaces, or engaging in shared interests e.g. playing a game of football. To achieve this, all patients should be aware of the name and role of the staff member observing them, and the range of activities available within their care environment.

Every period of nursing care should include a comprehensive evaluation of the patient's mental state and underlying issues, followed by the implementation of appropriate interventions for example, crisis management, positive behaviour support plans, MDT working. Risk assessment is central to all of these elements and is a key part of the nursing role. Safewards is an evidence-based intervention designed to minimise restriction conflict in mental health settings by focussing on ten key areas; these include fostering positive interactions, providing reassurance, employing de-escalation techniques, delivering bad news sensitively, and using calm communication with patients in crisis (Bowers, 2014). In a single-blinded cluster randomised controlled trial across fifteen hospitals, the implementation of Safewards resulted in a 15 per cent reduction in conflict rates and a 24 per cent decrease in containment measures, highlighting the importance of meaningful engagement of the nursing team (Bowers, 2015). Unfortunately, despite the best efforts of nurses and the broader multidisciplinary team to foster supportive and therapeutic environments, there are some instances when more restrictive interventions become necessary to keep patients and others safe. This may include administration of involuntary treatment, restricting of physical freedom (e.g. locking doors to prevent patients from leaving), and initiating Mental Health Act (2007) assessments.

Physical Restraint and Seclusion in Mental Health Settings

If patients pose immediate risks to the physical safety of themselves or others, the use of physical restraint and/or seclusion may also be deemed necessary. In such circumstances it is essential that nurses also do as much as possible to uphold the patient's human rights (Human Rights Act, 1998), and use these interventions judiciously by adhering to established guidelines and regularly reassessing the necessity for such measures as the patient's presentation evolves, (Care Act, 2014). Physical restraint in mental health settings involves using direct physical contact to prevent or restrict a patient's movement when other de-escalation techniques have failed. It is vital that the level of restraint being used is proportionate to the assessed risk of harm, and that health professionals who may be involved in physical restraint have access to approved training and relevant hospital policies. This is particularly pertinent for mental health nurses, who are typically expected to lead a physical restraint and ensure that it is applied for the shortest duration necessary. Nurses are also responsible for monitoring the patient's physical health during a restraint, tailoring care plans to accommodate an individual's movement capabilities and ensuring that thorough documentation is completed. At an appropriate time after the use of physical restraint, debriefing is also important (for both staff members and the patient) to reflect on the experience, and improve future practice, (Department of Health, 1983).

Seclusion involves the supervised confinement of a patient in a locked room to manage the risks associated with severe behavioural disturbance; it should never been use punitively and only considered when all other measures have been attempted and found inadequate. Guidance for seclusion rooms emphasise the importance of safety and functionality to ensure the well-being of the patient being secluded. Key requirements include the elimination of potential safety hazards, externally controlled heating and air conditioning and the provision of communication with staff e.g. via an intercom. The design of seclusion rooms should also eliminate potential blind spots so that the patient can be kept under continuous observation, allowing for prompt intervention if necessary. Seclusion should be regarded as a means of stabilising the patient so that appropriate therapeutic interventions can resume once the immediate risk has been mitigated. Proper protocols and oversight must therefore be maintained during seclusion to safeguard the dignity and human rights of the patient, (Department of Health, 1983).

Nurses play a key role throughout the seclusion process. They are usually present with the patient when a period of seclusion begins, facilitating a seamless handover to relevant medical professional and thorough/timely documentation. Mental health nurses are also responsible for creating a comprehensive seclusion care plan that addresses the patient's risks, dietary/fluid/hygiene needs, and the criteria being used for terminating seclusion as soon as possible. To ensure safety, nurses must ensure that patients in seclusion are under continuous enhanced observation by appropriately skilled staff and that the patient's presentation and status is documented every 15 minutes. After two hours of seclusion, two nurses (one of whom was not part of the initial seclusion decision) should also review the patient's risk assessment, daily living activities, and medication management. The nursing team must ensure that any policies related to the use of seclusion are adhered to and obtain medical confirmation before terminating seclusion. When a decision is made to terminate a period of seclusion, nurses need to ensure that all relevant documentation has been completed and (when appropriate) facilitate a debrief with the patient and staff involved.

Restrictive practices in healthcare serve to manage the risk of harm and should be used as a last resort, (Lawrence, 2025). The Care Quality Commission, (CQC, 2017) emphasises the importance of minimising such interventions, including physical restraint and seclusion, urging healthcare providers to adopt tailored approaches rather than a one-size-fits-all strategy. Each patient should receive a personalised care plan that addresses their unique needs and circumstances, thereby promoting safety while respecting their individual rights and dignity. This individualised approach is essential for reducing reliance on restrictive measures and fostering a more therapeutic care approach, (CQC, 2017).

Whilst the use of restrictive practices can make it challenging for mental health nurses to develop and maintain therapeutic relationships with their patients, advocacy can reduce the potential barriers by ensuring that patients are aware of their rights and able to have their voice heard. Nurses are the professional group most likely to be responsible for ensuring that, under s132 Mental Health Act 1983 (amended 2007), reasonable steps have been taken to ensure that detained patients are aware of their rights. This may require more than one attempt (e.g. if the patient is initially too distressed to process this information), or the provision of information in alternative formats (e.g. translated/easy-read versions). The advocacy role that nurses hold also extends to supporting patients' carers to engage in positive interactions, facilitate coping strategies, and nurture resilience. Indeed, the Carer's Trust (n.d.) have identified six key standards that are central to the nursing role:

- Identifying carers and their role as soon as possible in the person's care journey.
- Using expertise to engage with carers.
- Ensuring that policy and protocols are in place around information sharing.
- Ensuring that defined posts for carers are in place.
- Ensuring that a carer introduction is available.
- Making a range of carer services available.

Depending on the patient's circumstances, mental health nurses may also be involved in providing psychoeducation, relapse prevention, and realistic goal settings with carers. Patient confidentiality should not be a barrier to providing general information about which services are available or receiving information and updates from carers.

Detained patients should also be aware that they may have a right to an Independent Mental Health Advocate (IMHA); these are specially trained people, independent to the detaining authority, who can support patients by ensuring that their rights are upheld. IMHAs also have an important role in ensuring that the patient's views and wishes are represented in meetings and/ or when clinical decision making happens.

Nursing and Medication Management

Historically, biological models of illness have been given primacy in the treatment of mental disorders and medication is often a first line treatment for people experiencing serious mental illness. Although advances in non-pharmacological treatments mean that medication is now only regarded as one of a range of evidence-based interventions, medication monitoring, and interventions to improve concordance are still significant parts of mental health nursing treatment plans.

Insight refers to a patient's ability to recognise their symptoms or understand why other people may be concerned about them. As such, people with no insight or where insight is limited are more likely to want to discontinue medication abruptly against medical advice, (Novick et al., 2015). To support this patient sub-population, psychoeducation is augmented in the patient's care plan with the aim of developing to increase the patient's insight, and thereby concordance with medication, by providing individuals with appropriate information and support, for them to explore their own symptom attributions and experiences of mental distress. This may include understanding the patient's distress using the stress-vulnerability model, timelines, and early warning sign recognition, usually resulting in the coproduction of a relapse prevention/staying well plan.

Other ways that mental health nurses can facilitate medication concordance is through prompting/encouraging patients to receive their medication at regular times, delivering medication, and management of so-called "as required" medications (understanding the frequency that these medications are used may give an indication of the severity of the patient's symptoms). Mental health nurses are well placed to assess how patients respond to medication administration and therefore the likelihood that they will remain concordant in less restrictive environments. Some care environments, for example, facilitate patients to self-medicate i.e. giving patients responsibility for administering their own medications independently.

Under the provisions of the Mental Health Act 1983 (amended 2007), some patients in hospital can be compelled to accept treatment against their wishes. One of the most restrictive roles undertaken by mental health nurses is therefore enforcing medication administration e.g. by administering rapid tranquilisation or long-acting injections (often referred to as depot injections/depots) under physical restraint. This practice is likely to be traumatic for patients and nurses alike and should therefore only be performed when less restrictive options have been exhausted. In light of this, some mental health nurses have called for a right to conscientiously object from this practice, (Gadsby and McKeown, 2021).

Concordance with mental health medications may also be reduced by the impact of unpleasant side effects, which in some circumstances may constitute a form of iatrogenic harm. Commonly experienced side effects of antipsychotic medications, for example, include drowsiness, extra-pyramidal side effects (e.g. stiffness, tremor) and increased risk of metabolic syndrome. Metabolic syndrome is an umbrella term for a range of biological changes (including hypertension, dyslipidaemia, abdominal obesity, and hyperglycaemia) which significantly increase cardiovascular risk. As such, mental health nurses need to ensure that patients receive appropriate physical health monitoring depending on the medication they are taking, and any comorbid physical health conditions and treatments. This is particularly important when new medications are initiated, or when doses of existing medications are altered. National guidelines therefore recommend that all patients prescribed antipsychotic medications are offered a baseline physical health assessment, including physical observations (blood pressure, heart rate, BMI, waist circumference) and an electrocardiogram (ECG) (NICE, 2014).

Whilst taking psychiatric medications, individuals are also likely to need on-going physical health monitoring e.g. patients taking Olanzapine should have their BMI monitored and six-monthly blood tests, patients taking lithium should receive three monthly monitoring of lithium levels, thyroid, and kidney function. However, since the degree and frequency of required monitoring will depend on both patient- and medication-specific factors, coordinating this requires expert care planning as well as an individualised and patient-centred approach. In order to respond appropriately to side effects, mental health nurses require expert knowledge of psychiatric medications as well as national guidelines and should supplement their observations using validated screening and monitoring tools for example, LUNSERS, (Liverpool University Neuroleptic Side Effect Rating Scale), (Day et al., 1995). Since some of the potential side effects of psychiatric medications are commonly associated with embarrassment or stigma e.g. sexual dysfunction, mental health nurses also need to be skilled communicators in order to ensure that their patients receive appropriate medication monitoring.

Although usually rarer, some mental health medications are also linked to potentially fatal side effects. Clozapine (an antipsychotic medication used primarily for treatment resistant schizophrenia), for example, is associated with an increased risk of pericarditis, agranulocytosis, and life-threatening gastrointestinal hypomotility. Mental health nurses therefore play an essential role in advising patients about these risks (including how to recognise when to seek urgent advice) and supporting them to access appropriate monitoring interventions e.g. attending phlebotomy appointments, recording frequency of bowel movements.

Individuals experiencing mental distress may find it harder to engage with mainstream health services and health promoting behaviours. Addressing this has been identified as a public health priority (Department of Health and Social Care, 2023) given that people with serious mental illness are at an increased risk of morbidity and premature death (Chesney, Goodwin and Fazel, 2014). As such, GP practices are encouraged to keep up-to-date registers of people with severe mental illness and their:

- Alcohol consumption
- Blood glucose or HbA1c
- Blood pressure
- Body mass index (BMI)
- Lipid profile
- Smoking status.

Mental health nurses also have a vital role in promoting positive health behaviours and can support their patients with severe mental illness by helping them to register with a General Practitioner (GP), access universal screening programmes, and attend planed appointments with other health specialists e.g. dieticians, dentists, opticians, diabetes nurses. Mental health nurses are also well placed to provide patients with health promotion themselves e.g. advice regarding smoking cessation, sleep hygiene, healthy eating, harm minimisation.

Conclusion

This chapter gives a broad overview of the key roles and responsibilities of mental health nurses across different care settings; whilst there might be significant differences in the environments where care is provided, the guiding principles still apply. By closely monitoring patients and providing timely interventions, nurses can minimise the need for restrictive measures. This chapter also demonstrates that nurses are key to the delivery of mental health care, the availability of appropriate medical treatment and upholding patient rights by ensuring that care is provided in the least restrictive way.

References

Allen, D. (2020). A nurse's guide to cognitive behaviour therapy. *Nursing Standard.* 35(1): 35–37. doi: 10.7748/ns.35.1.35.s15

Birchwood, M., Spencer, E., and McGovern, D. (2000). Schizophrenia: early warning signs. *Advances in Psychiatric Treatment.* 6(2): 93–101. doi:10.1192/apt.6.2.93

Bowers, L. (2014). Safewards: a new model of conflict and containment on psychiatric wards. *Journal of Psychiatric and Mental Health Nursing.* 21(6). doi: 10.1111/jpm.12129

Bowers, L., James, K., Quirk, A., et al. (2015). Reducing conflict and containment rates on acute psychiatric wards: the safewards cluster randomises controlled trial. *International Journal of Nursing Studies.* 52(9). doi: 10.1016/j.ijnurstu.2015.05.001

Brennan, G. (2023). Stress vulnerability model of serious mental illness. In Gamble, C., and Brennan, G. (eds) *Working with serious mental illness. A manual for clinical practice* (3rd ed.). Elsevier (chapter 3).

Care Act. (2014). *Promoting individual wellbeing.* Available at www.legislation.gov.uk/ukpga/2014/23/section/1 [Accessed 25 March 2025].

Care Quality Commission (CQC). (2017). *Mental Health Act, A focus on restrictive intervention reduction programmes in inpatient mental health services.* Available at www.cqc.org.uk/publications/themed-work/mental-health-act-restrictive-intervention-reduction-programmes [Accessed 25 March 2025].

Carer's Trust. (n.d.). *The triangle of care.* Available at https://carers.org/triangle-of-care/the-triangle-of-care [Accessed 27 March 2025].

Chesney, E., Goodwin, G. M., and Fazel, S. (2014). Risks of all-cause mortality in mental disorders: a meta-review. *World Psychiatry.* 13(2): 153–160. doi: 10.1002/wps.20128

Cutler, N. A., Sim, J., Halcomb, E., Moxham, L., and Stephens, M. (2020). Nurses' influence on consumers' experience of safety in acute mental health units: a qualitative study. *Journal of Clinical Nursing.* 29(21–22). doi: 10.1111/jocn.15480#

Day, J. C., Wood, G., Dewey, M., and Bentall, R. P. (1995). A self-rating scale for measuring neuroleptic side-effects. *British Journal of Psychiatry.* 166(5): 650–653. doi: 10.1192/bjp.166.5.650

Department of Health. (1983). *Mental Health Act, Code of Practice. Physical restraint.* Available at www.publishing.service.gov.uk [Accessed 25 March 2025].

Department of Health. (1983). *Mental Health Act, Code of Practice. Seclusion.* Available at www.publishing.service.gov.uk [Accessed 25 March 2025].

d'Ettorre, G., Pellicani, V., Mazzotta, M., et al. (2018). Preventing and managing workplace violence against healthcare workers in Emergency Departments. *Health Professions.* 89(4-s). doi: 10.23750/abm.v89i4-S.7113

Department of Health and Social Care. (2023). *Major conditions strategy: case for change and our strategic framework.* Available at www.GOV.UK [Accessed 25 March 2025].

Gadsby, J., and McKeown, M. (2021). Mental health nursing and conscientious objection to forced pharmaceutical intervention. *Nursing Philosophy.* 22(4). doi: 10.1111/nup.12369

Gilburt, H., and Mallorie, S. (2024). *Mental health 360.* King's Fund. Available at www.kingsfund.org.uk/insight-and-analysis/long-reads/mental-health-360 [Accessed 29 March 2025].

Hallett, N., and Dickens, G. G. (2015). De-escalation: a survey of clinical staff in a secure mental health inpatient service. *International Journal of Mental Health Nursing.* 24(4). doi: 10.1111/inm.12136

Hurley, J., Lakeman, R., Linsley, P., et al. (2022). Utilizing the mental health nursing workforce: a scoping review of mental health nursing clinical roles and identities. *International Journal of Mental Health Nursing.* 31(4). doi: 10.1111/inm.12983

Jerome, L., McNamee, P., Abdel-Halim., N., Elliot, K., and Woods, J. (2023). Solution-focused approaches in adult mental health research: a conceptual literature review and narrative synthesis. *Frontiers in Psychiatry.* doi: 10.3389/fpsyt.2023.1068006

Lawrence, D. (2025). *Restrictive practices in secure mental health services.* Cardiff Metropolitan University, https://figshare.cardiffmet.ac.uk/articles/thesis/Restrictive_practices_in_secure_mental_health_services/28430036?file=52419230.

López-López, J. A., Davies, S. R., Caldwell, D. M., et al. (2019). The process and delivery of CBT for depression in adults: a systematic review and network meta-analysis. *Psychological Medicine.* 49(12): 1937–1947. doi: 10.1017/S003329171900120X

Marland, G., McNay, L., and Fleming, M. (2011). Using timelines as part of recovery – focused practice in psychosis. *Journal of Psychiatric and Mental Health Nursing.* 18(10): 869–877.

Mental Health UK. (2018). *The stress bucket.* Available at https://mentalhealth-uk.org/blog/the-stress-bucket/ [Accessed 25 March 2025].

Miller, W. R. (2023). The evolution of motivational interviewing. *Behavioural and Cognitive Psychology.* 51(6): 1–17.

Miller, W. R., and Rollnick, S. (2013). *Motivational interviewing: helping people to change* (3rd ed.). Guilford Press.

Miller, W. R., and Rollnick, S. (2013). *Motivational interviewing: helping people to change* (3rd ed.). Guilford Press.

National Institute for Health and Care Excellence (NICE). (2014). *Psychosis and schizophrenia in adults: prevention and management.* Available at www.nice.org.uk/guidance/cg178 [Accessed 29 March 2025].

National Institute for Health and Care Excellence (NICE). (2015). *Violence and aggression: short-term management in mental health, health and community settings.* Available at www.nice.org.uk/guidance/ng10 [Accessed 24 March 2025].

New Economics Foundation (NEF). (2008). *Five ways to wellbeing.* London: NEF.

NHS. (n.d.). *Better Health every mind matters: Reframing unhelpful thoughts.* Available at www.nhs.uk/every-mind-matters/mental-wellbeing-tips/self-help-cbt-techniques/reframing-unhelpful-thoughts/#cycle [Accessed 25 March 2025].

NHS England. (2024). *Culture of care standards for mental health inpatient services.* Available at www.england.nhs.uk/long-read/culture-of-care-standards-for-mental-health-inpatient-services/ [Accessed 25 March 2025].

Novick, D., Montgomery, W., Treuer, T., et al. (2015). Relationship of insight with medication adherence and impact on outcomes in patients with schizophrenia and bipolar disorder: results from a 1-year European outpatient observational study. *BMC Psychiatry.* 5(15). doi: 10.1186/s12888-015-0560-4

Nursing and Midwifery Council (NMC). (2018). *Future nurse: standards of proficiency for registered nurses.* Available at www.future-nurse-proficiencies.pdf [Accessed 25 March 2025].

Proudlock, S., and Sanghvi, S. (2017). Using solution-focused approaches (chapter 41, pp. 453–463). In Chambers, M. (ed) *Psychiatric and mental health nursing. The craft of caring* (3rd ed.). Oxon: Routledge.

Stephenson, L., Gergel, T., Owen, G., et al. (2019). *The future of advanced decision making in the Mental Health Act.* King's College London. Available at www.adm-mental-health-act.pdf [Accessed 25 March 2025].

The Human Rights Act (HRA). (1998). *The convention rights.* Available at www.legislation.gov.uk [Accessed 21 March 2025].

Veitch, P., Strong, L., and Armstrong, N. (2017). Assertive outreach (Chapter 56). In Chambers, M. (ed) *Psychiatric and mental health nursing. The craft of caring.* (3rd ed.). Oxon: Routledge.

Zubin, J., and Spring, B. (1977). Vulnerability: a new view of schizophrenia. *Journal of Abnormal Psychology.* 86: 260–266.

6   Exploring Community Mental Health Services

Barbara Deacon-Hedges and Helen Rees

Introduction

The National Collaborating Centre for Mental Health, (2021), encourages those working within mental healthcare to adopt a broad definition of the word "community". This includes recognising that individuals may belong to many different communities at the same time e.g. occupation, religion, and interests (National Collaborating Centre for Mental Health, 2021), and that the social connections which underpin communities can be an important source of strength and resilience, (Fone et al., 2014). This is especially pertinent to people with serious mental illness who are not only at increased risk of social isolation but may experience social isolation as a precipitating factor for relapse, (Majmudar et al., 2022). The majority of mental healthcare is delivered by community mental health services. It is estimated that 3.58 million people in England had contact with either NHS mental health, learning disability or autism services between 2022 and 2023, (NHS England Digital, 2024). This figure is likely to be an underestimate since it does not include contact with non-NHS mental health services, for example those provided by the private and voluntary sectors.

In addition to building resilience, the existence of community mental health services promotes the guiding principles of the Mental Health Act Code of Practice e.g. *Least restrictive option and maximising independence,* (Department of Health, 2015, p23). Upholding this principle requires mental health practitioners to ensure that they give preference to interventions that do not involve detention and/or compulsion. It also means that practitioners need to be person-centred (considering the patient's individualised needs) and ensure that any restrictions imposed on patients are enforced for the shortest amount of time possible. Achieving this requires a complicated system of community-based interventions, provided by statutory, voluntary, and charitable organisations (in collaboration with the patient's family and support network). This chapter will outline the role played by community mental health services, the underpinning guidance/policies supporting these services and the value of community mental health services in supporting a "person's rights and freedom of action", (Department of Health, 2015, p23). It will also encourage the reader to consider the wider context of individuals receiving mental health services (and the difference they can make to health outcomes) by incorporating their voice and the voices of those who care for them.

Background

The development of community mental healthcare in the UK reflects changing views on mental illness/detention/human rights, the development of new treatments and concerns around the negative effects of institutionalisation. Understanding the role that community mental health

DOI: 10.4324/9781003635543-7

services play therefore requires an awareness of the political, theoretical, economic, and social landscape that influenced the current model of provision. Whilst the outpatient provision of psychiatric care was enshrined in law as early as the Mental Treatment Act (1930), it was not until the 1950s that Victorian-style mental health asylums started to close in an attempt to deinstitutionalise people with serious mental illness (Burns, 2020). Activists from the survivor movement and critical psychiatry, (Turner, 2015) also proposed that the singular medical model of mental illness was ineffective in supporting people experiencing mental distress, leading to mainstream acceptance of the bio-psycho-social-spiritual model of mental illness, (Wade and Halligan, 2017). This model is underpinned by the stress-vulnerability model, (Engel, 1977), which states that mental illnesses can be attributed to the interaction between an individual's vulnerabilities (e.g. having a strong family history of mental illness), stressors (e.g. bereavement, financial hardship, relationship breakdown), and resilience. Adopting this model requires mental health practitioners to understand patients within their wider context, including their social connections and communities. The evolving provision of community mental health services has been further influenced by the recovery movement, which argues against the premise that the only objective of mental healthcare is the elimination of symptoms of mental illness, (Johansson and Holmes, 2023). Instead, the movement promotes a holistic, person-centred approach based on the following two principles, (Fortune et al., 2015):

1. It is possible to recover from a mental health condition.
2. The most effective recovery is patient-directed.

Over time, policy makers have continued to acknowledge the importance of providing community mental healthcare for patients in recovery. In 1971, for example, the Department of Health and Social Security gave local authorities the responsibility of supporting individuals discharged from hospital, leading to the development of supported living, day services and increased access to community mental health practitioners, (Department of Health and Social Security, 1971).

Whilst perceptions of mental illness and mental health stigma have changed over time, the policy and legal frameworks underpinning community mental healthcare have arguably not always been founded on social inclusion and the reduction of discrimination/coercion. It is therefore important to acknowledge that whilst community mental health services play an essential role in risk management, they can be perceived as overly restrictive: this is exemplified by some of the debates surrounding Community Treatment Orders, (Mental Health Act, 1983), (Dawson, 2023). The King's Fund (2015), also suggests that the provision of additional resources to community mental health services has been at the expense of inpatient services, resulting in fewer inpatient practitioners and reduced availability of inpatient beds.

Mental Health Service Provision – the Current Context

The provision of community mental healthcare is a key public health issue: the last Adult Psychiatry Morbidity Survey, (NHS England (2016), for example, found that in any given week in England, approximately 1 in 6 adults report experiencing symptoms of common mental health problems. This is likely to be an underestimate given that there has been a significant increase in referrals to mental health services since this survey was conducted, (NHS Digital, 2024). It is also estimated that 1 in 5 children and young people have a probable mental disorder, (NHS England, 2023). Given the scale of this issue, there is a recognised need for mental health services to be proactive and cost-effective. NHS England therefore currently sets waiting time standards for two adult community mental health services: NHS talking therapies, and early intervention in psychosis teams (Department of Health and Social Care, 2014). The focus on waiting times reflects the NHS plans to achieve timely access, and proactive intervention, reflecting the importance of early intervention and recovery models, (Department of Health and Social Care, 2023). However, at the time of writing, the waiting time standards do not exist for other community mental health services e.g. crisis services and community mental health teams, which puts some people experiencing mental health challenges at increased risk of delayed treatment, poorer health outcomes, and compulsory detention under the Mental Health Act, (1983).

Unfortunately, there are frequent reports of people experiencing lack of resources and a fragmented approach when trying to access community mental health services, (Department of Health and Social Care, 2023). There have been a number of government policies aimed at tackling this: the NHS Long Term Plan, (Department of Health and Social Care, 2014), the NHS Mental Health Implementation Plan (NHS England, 2019) and the Major Conditions Strategy, (Department of Health and Social Care, 2023), for example, all set out how the NHS will develop/ integrate models of community care and provide necessary funding and support. Central to these policies are increased access to psychological therapies, improvements in physical care for people with serious mental illness, a commitment to social prescribing, and providing trauma informed care. This will be achieved through integrated care systems (ICS), bringing together health and care organisations in a particular geographical area (serving between 600'000 and a million people) to work together more closely and provide joined-up care, (Charles, 2022; NHS England, 2022). As well as including NHS organisations, this alliance may include social care providers, voluntary organisations, community groups, social enterprises, and others with a role in improving the health and wellbeing of local people (such as education, housing, employment, or police and fire services). Whilst ICS are at an early stage of development, they are likely to be key for making multi-agency commissioning decisions e.g. regarding health and social care support systems and supported housing, (The King's Fund 2022).

The King's Fund (2024), highlights that there are patchy services for mental health, especially for young people and autism services, and a focus on immediate needs over long term planning. The aim of the NHS Long Term Plan, (NHS England, 2019) is therefore to modernise community health services to ensure a whole-person, whole-population approach aligned to Primary Care Networks. Primary Care Networks aim to connect and support primary care leaders to improve the health and wellbeing of communities (with a heavy influence on neighbourhoods, place and system level working), The King's Fund (2020).

The Role of Community Mental Health Care in Discharge Planning

When a patient is admitted to hospital for a mental health problem, discharge planning should start as soon as possible and be a collaborative process between health professionals, patients and the patient's family/support network, (The Department of Health and Social Care, 2024). This should include an individual assessment of the patient's needs and ensuring that community mental health services are in place if required, (NHS England, 2024). Indeed, Section 117 of the Mental Health Act (1983) places a statutory duty on local authorities to provide aftercare for people detained under some sections of the Act. In addition to the provision of mental health services, discharge planning should involve supporting patients to access any state benefits they are entitled to, identifying appropriate accommodation, and arranging access to meaningful activity. While decision-making responsibility for funding these interventions typically sits with senior commissioning managers in both NHS and local authority organisations, it is important to recognise that the care planning, review, and application for Section 117 funding is often undertaken by health and social care practitioners.

Finances

Since some state benefits are stopped when patients are admitted to hospital, access to money can be a significant source of stress for people being discharged from psychiatric hospitals. The symptoms of mental illness can also make it more difficult for someone to access the state benefits they are entitled to and comply with the rules required to continue receiving them e.g. attending appointments (Smith, 2024). It is therefore unsurprising that compared to the general population, mental health patients are at increased risk of debt (Smith, 2024). Financial stress is also likely to perpetuate mental distress and put patients at increased risk of relapse. Asking about money concerns is therefore an essential part of a holistic assessment.

- It is important that unemployed patients are supported to contact the Department for Work and Pensions (DWP) when they are unwell.
- Mental health staff should advocate for patients and support them to work with DWP to provide a trusted contact.
- Carers should also be supported to apply for any state benefits they are entitled to (to support the extra costs associated with this role).
- Patients experiencing a mental health crisis may be eligible to apply for the "breathing space scheme" (HM Treasury, 2023). This is designed to protect those in crisis from accruing debt. NHS England have produced an eLearning module about the breathing space scheme for mental health professionals.
- People with severe mental illness may be eligible for Personal Independence Payments (PIP), Gov UK (n.d.). This is a non-means tested benefit, designed to support people with the extra living costs associated with having a long-term disability.
- Supporting someone to apply for state benefits may be an essential part of discharge planning. Although this is often considered to be the responsibility of an occupational therapist or social worker, all mental health staff should have the skills to provide support in this area.

Accommodation

If a patient wishes to return to their own accommodation after an admission to psychiatric hospital, there are several areas of support that need to be considered. Firstly, a visit to the property can help mental health professionals to ascertain what support the individual may need to make the property safe. Mental illness can impact on all activities of daily living so observing someone in their own environment can also help to determine if they are able to meet needs such as nutrition, self-care, and sleep. A care assessment carried out by the local authority can determine if someone is eligible for support with their daily living e.g. home alterations, childcare, carer services, and support with cleaning. Although care assessments are free, individuals may be expected to contribute to the cost of the interventions recommended by social services depending on their individual circumstances (NHS, n.d.). Patients who have difficulties managing their utility services may accrue debt or be cut off during a period of hospitalisation and should therefore be encouraged to join the priority services register; the benefits of this include being able to select your preferred contact method and nominate a trusted individual for utility companies to communicate with, (PSR, n.d.).

There are alternative accommodation options for patients who do not own or lease their own properties. Short term options include rehabilitation placements or supported accommodation as part of Section 117 aftercare, (Mental Health Act, 1983). These are generally staffed and may support patients with their activities of daily living. However, since the qualifications/availability of staff and level of support offered varies between different service providers, knowing what will be provided upon discharge is likely to be important information for the mental health tribunal to consider when deciding whether a patient can be discharged safely from detention. A facilities report is a standardised way for sharing this information. It is particularly important to provide feedback from any leave trials to staffed accommodation. This should include information such as mental state, concordance with care, and interaction with staff and other people living in the accommodation.

Longer term accommodation options include care homes and residential homes. These are usually considered for patients with intractable mental disorders or those with an organic/progressive nature and are frequently facilitated under deprivation of liberty frameworks, (Mental Capacity Act, 2005). Care homes and residential homes usually offer a high level of support to patients e.g. permanent availability of trained staff.

Regardless of the patient's needs, upholding the least restrictive principle of the Act requires those involved in their care to work collaboratively to ensure that a safe and suitable discharge destination is identified in timely manner. Achieving this also requires effective communication within/between teams, clear care planning and unambiguity regarding who is responsible for the different roles involved in the patient's discharge.

NHS Community Mental Health Services

Since engaging with community mental health services can build resilience and reduce the likelihood of hospital detention for people experiencing mental distress, evaluating the likelihood that patients will make themselves available for appointments and engage with treatment is an extremely important component of risk formulation. It is therefore essential that those giving evidence to the tribunal are familiar with what services are available in the community and what has been done to develop a therapeutic relationship with the patient to date (in order to form a view about the likelihood of disengagement). Since the immediate period following inpatient discharge is associated with elevated risk, it is also vital that inpatient and community mental health services work together and share information in order to reduce the possibility of a fragmented transition between services at the point of discharge, (Nuffield Trust, 2024). Discharging patients in a coordinated manner also allows community mental health services to facilitate a 72-hour post discharge health check as recommended by the Department of Health and Social Care (2024).

Primary Mental Health Services

In the general population, most people experiencing mental health challenges are managed by services within primary care and offered interventions provided by General Practitioners, mental health practitioners and registered mental health nurses e.g. talking therapies for common mental disorders. Primary care services also typically offer a range of wellbeing activities such as walking groups, leisure activities, and occupational activities, (Royal College of Psychiatrists, 2021) which can be accessed through social prescribing. Since they have oversight of all the services involved in an individual's care, primary care providers also play an important role in safeguarding vulnerable patients (and those around them) and referring patients to secondary mental health services where appropriate.

Secondary Mental Health Services

Although the provision of secondary mental health care is largely determined by individual need, the accessibility of specific services is based on a variety of factors including the patient's demographic data, diagnostic criteria and symptom severity. Commissioning decisions are also not universal meaning that it is not possible to guarantee which interventions are available regionally. The next part of this chapter therefore outlines the main forms of community support available from NHS secondary mental health providers.

Home treatment and crisis care teams provide immediate care to patients experiencing mental health challenges on a time-limited/short-term basis for rehabilitation, reablement and recovery at home, (HM Government, 2014). Patients who are in crisis and already known to secondary mental health services typically have access to crisis care teams 24 hours a day and 7 days a week, (HM Government, 2014). Similarly, home treatment teams support patients at increased risk of relapse/death by suicide (Department of Health and Social Care, 2024) by providing medication management/supervision, intensive mental state/risk monitoring, and short-term psychosocial interventions. Both crisis and home treatment teams also have a pivotal role in safeguarding, gatekeeping inpatient admissions and arranging Mental Health Act assessments for patients who meet the statutory criteria for hospital detention.

Community or local mental health teams (CMHTs / LMHTs) see the majority of patients who require longer-term support from secondary mental health services. These patients are typically referred when their mental health needs can no longer be managed within primary care; the referral criteria for CMHTs are not diagnosis-specific and the frequency of appointments offered will depend upon the needs of the individual. Some community mental health teams also have access to day centre facilities which are designed to build resilience and support patients at risk of deterioration (by providing meaningful activity, increased contact with health professionals and a structured/safe way to spend the day). Community mental health teams comprise psychiatrists, psychologists, registered mental health nurses, support workers, social workers and occupational therapists. Many teams also employ peer support workers to share their lived experience of living with a mental disorder; there is evidence that peer support instils hope, improves resilience and encourages patients to take responsibility for managing their condition, (NHS England, 2023). All community mental health services offer a range of pharmacological and non-pharmacological interventions: these include medication proscribing/management, relapse prevention, budgeting support, advanced care planning, supporting access to meaningful activity, family interventions, safeguarding, and talking therapies. Most of these are completed without compulsion and therefore rely on patients accessing and engaging with services by choice.

Assertive Outreach Teams (AOT) work with patients who are considered "difficult to engage" i.e. those who consistently avoid contact with mental health services leading to deterioration in their mental health, (NHS England, 2024). It does this by reducing some of the barriers that prevent people with serious mental illness from engaging (e.g. by offering home visits) as well as providing a similar range of interventions to CMHTs. AOT requires more resources to achieve its aims but is still deemed to be cost-effective by reducing the burden on crisis support teams and need for hospital admissions. It is important to note that the concept of "difficult to engage" has been challenged by people with experience of services who have highlighted that disengagement is frequently due to barriers, a history of poor service, and difficulties in accessing services rather than a wish not to engage with care that is offered.

CMHTs and AOT accept patients with a range of diagnoses. However, some mental disorders require such specific interventions that commissioners agree to fund specialist services. These may include services for people with dual diagnosis, first episode psychosis, eating disorders, drug and alcohol misuse, personality disorders, and neurodevelopmental disorders. These services usually have more rigid referral criteria to ensure that resources are used expeditiously. Mental health services that include age in their eligibility criteria include children and young person services (sometimes referred to as CAMHS) and older adult teams. These services benefit patients by taking into account the impact of age on biological, social, and psychological milestones. As well as having specialist knowledge of the mental disorders which commonly affect younger/older people, these teams also work closely with the partner agencies most likely to be involved with their patients e.g. schools, looked after children services and social care services. Unfortunately, patients known to CAMHS often find the transition to adult services distressing; this usually happens when patients turn 18 years old, which is a time of significant uncertainty for many people e.g. starting university, learning to drive, moving away from home. In recognition of this, and the NHS Long Term Plan, (NHS England, 2019), some secondary mental health service providers now provide a 0-25 service for children and young people, and have removed the age barriers for general adult community mental health services.

Telemental Health Services

Some community mental health services are now provided over telephone or video services; this allows an individual to receive mental health care remotely. Whilst this is a fairly new way of working in England, it is an established way of working in some countries where the geographical location of services means that it is not practical for all contact to be done face to face. The flexibility of offering telemental health means that people may not need to take time out of education or employment and has shown to have similar outcomes as face-to-face appointments for some people (Sugarman, 2023). It is important that patient preference, severity of illness and risk formulation are considered when making the decision of what format to provide care. The digital divide means that some people face barriers in accessing telemental heath, such as not having access to equipment that allows engagement, or not having a quite private space available to take the appointment. It is important that the decision is not based on stereotypes, for instance assuming that young people would prefer telemental health, 8% of children aged 5–15 in the UK do not have access to an internet enabled computer, laptop or net book at home (UNICEF, 2021).

Coordination of Community Care

As already stated, many different teams, agencies and organisations can be involved in providing care to a person experiencing serious mental illness. In recognition of this, continuity, coordination and organisation of patient's care was previously overseen by a framework known as the Care Programme Approach (CPA). However, the use of CPA as a gatekeeper to care coordination was criticised for inconsistency (due to variability in the accessibility criteria of different teams and services) (NHS England, 2022). This has led to services moving away from the CPA approach and adopting alternative frameworks in order to provide patients with severe mental illness with access to high-quality, person-centred care planning and implementation (NHS England, 2022). An example of this is the DIALOG framework that is designed to provide a structure to ensuring care is focused on the needs identified by the individual receiving that care, (Priebe, McCabe and Bullencamp, 2007).

Support for Carers

It is essential that community mental health services consider those who provide patients with informal care and support (e.g. family members, partners, friends) as key members of the interprofessional team. The Carers Trust, (2023), for example, describes the therapeutic alliance between patients, carers, and professionals as the triangle of care. It is therefore essential that community mental health services develop good channels of communication with their patients' support networks and consider the needs of carers. It is also vital that the views of carers are sought/considered when making important clinical decisions; this is not only a legal duty in the case of Nearest Relatives (Mental Health Act, 1983) but also a way of increasing the likelihood that a care plan is effective/successful. Although sharing information with carers can result in ethical/legal dilemmas, the Royal College of Psychiatrists (2017) is clear that confidentiality should not be used as a barrier to exclude carers wherever possible. It is therefore important that mental health professionals involved in such decision making have access to regular clinical supervision and multidisciplinary team discussions.

Although a patient's support network can make a significant contribution to recovery from serious mental illness (The Carers Trust, 2023), burnout, poor physical health and an increased risk of mental illness are reported by carers of people with serious mental illness, see Box 6.1, (Sanders, 2020). It is therefore important that community mental health services provide resilience building support for individuals with caring responsibilities. This could be achieved in a variety of ways including support groups, support to access carer-based benefits, talking therapies, and family interventions.

Wider Services

The majority of interventions aiming to improve mental wellbeing are provided by organisations outside of formal mental health services. Examples of these interventions provided by the voluntary and third sector include:

- Welfare benefits and other support from the Department of Work and Pensions
- Local advice and support agencies such as Citizen Advice Bureau
- Food banks
- Gym and leisure spaces
- Sports groups
- Community Cafés
- Drop In Centres.

As demonstrated in Box 6.2, these services are experienced as key to building resilience and reducing stressors that can negatively impact on mental wellbeing. It is important that community practitioners scope what is available in their local area and support patients accordingly.

Box 6.1 Carer view

"I am not recognised except to provide an alert system to services when something goes wrong and then they don't seem to act quickly. It may be the first they that have heard that X is unwell for a while, but I have been coping with it for weeks before I ring just in case he gets better. When I ring, I am at my end not at my beginning."

Box 6.2 Service user perspective

It is important to think widely about what community support is available and when service users told us what things in the community helps them stay well answers included:

- Walking groups
- The Returning to Work Group
- Men with Sheds
- Bollywood dancing
- Chair Pilates to stop falls
- Community Art
- Poetry Aloud
- Tai Chi
- Creative writing
- Water colouring
- Several language courses
- TRE (tension releasing exercises)
- Meditation.

Reasons that these services were helpful included:

- Makes me feel part of a community
- Gave me an interest "Men with Shed was great – it was us blokes fixing things and sharing skills'
- A chance to talk to others... 'and not about my problems'
- Support
- A bit of structure to my week
- Access to things like computers to look for work or training.

This demonstrates that finding out what interests and engages a person is the first step to thinking about community mental health support and regarding individuals as partners in their care.

This may include journey planning and travel safety work, sharing early warning signs with other services, anxiety management, exposure and accompanying individuals to attend whilst gradually building up independence skills.

Conclusion

This chapter provides an overview of the policy and funding structures that influence community mental health services, how they impact on local provision and how the use of local community resources can help people to stay mentally well in the community. The current range and availability of community services differs across the country in response to local need and funding e.g. services supporting isolated people in rural communities are likely to need a different approach to those providing the same interventions to people living in a busy city centre. Since the Covid-19 pandemic there is also a growing recognition that community and local links help people to maintain mental wellness. Skilled mental health practitioners will therefore need to know their local area and the services within it so that they can sign-post their patients (and their patient's carers) to appropriate interventions. In doing so they will support their patient's recovery by optimising their ability to stay well and independent in the community.

References

Burns, T. (2020). Community-based mental health care in Britain. *Consortium Psychiatricum* 1(2): 14–20. doi: 10.17650/2712-7672-2020-1-2-14-20

Charles, A. (2022). Integrated care systems explained. www.kingsfund.org.uk/insight-and-analysis/longreads/integrated-care-systems-explained [Accessed 14 November 2024].

Citizens Advice. https://midsuffolkcab.org.uk/about-us/history-of-citizens-advice/

Dawson, J. (2023). Compulsory community treatment. Is it the least restrictive alternative? Chapter 19. In: Kelly, B. D. and Donnelly, M. (eds) *Routledge Handbook of Mental Health Law*. Routledge.

Department of Health (2015). *Code of practice; Mental Health Act 1983*. London: The Stationary Office.

Department of Health and Social Care (2024). Discharge from mental health inpatient settings. www.gov.uk/government/publications/discharge-from-mental-health-inpatient-settings/discharge-from-mental-health-inpatient-settings [Accessed 23rd November 2024].

Department of Health and Social Care (2023). Major conditions strategy: case for change and out strategic framework. www.gov.uk/government/publications/major-conditions-strategy-case-for-change-and-our-strategic-framework/major-conditions-strategy-case-for-change-and-our-strategic-framework--2 [Accessed 4th November 2024].

Department of Health and Social Care (2014). Mental health services: achieving better access by 2020. www.gov.uk/government/publications/mental-health-services-achieving-better-access-by-2020 [Accessed 8th November 2024].

Department of Health and Social Security (1971). *Hospital services for the mentally ill*. London: Her Majesty's Stationary Office.

Engel, G. (1977). The need for a new medical model: a challenge for biomedicine. *Science* 196(4286): 129–136.

Fone, D., White, J., Farewell, D., Kelly, M., John, G. et al. (2014). Effect of neighbourhood deprivation and social cohesion on mental health inequality: a multilevel population-based longitudinal study. *Psychological Medicine* 44(11): 2449–2460.

Fortune, B., Bird, V., Chandler, R., Fox, J., Hennem, R., Larsen, J., Le Boutillier, C., Leamy, M., Macpherson, R., Williams, J., and Slade, M. (2015). Recovery for real. A summary of findings of the REFOCUS programme. www.researchintorecovery.com/files/Recovery%20for%20real%20-%20summary%20of%20REFOCUS%20programme_2.pdf [Accessed 27th November 2024].

Gov UK (n.d.). Personal Independence Payment (PIP). www.gov.uk/pip [Accessed 3rd November 2024].

HM Government (2014). Mental Health Crisis Care Concordat. Improving outcomes for people experiencing mental health crisis. https://assets.publishing.service.gov.uk/media/5a7c1ff0e5274a1f5cc75f09/36353_Mental_Health_Crisis_accessible.pdf [Accessed 11th November 2024].

HM Treasury (2023). Debt respite scheme (breathing space): guidance on mental health crisis breathing space. www.gov.uk/government/publications/debt-respite-scheme-breathing-space-guidance-on-mental-health-crisis-breathing-space [Accessed 21st November 2024].

Johansson, J. A., and Holmes, D. (2023). "Recovery" in mental health services, now and then: a poststructuralist examination of the despotic State machine's effects. *Nursing Inquiry* 31(3): 1–8. DOI: 10.1111/nin.12558

Majmudar, I. K., Mihalopoulos, C., Brijnath, B., Lim, M. H., Hall, N. Y., and Engel, L. (2022). The impact of loneliness and social isolation on health state utility values: a systematic literature review. *Quality Life*

Research 31(7): 1977–1997. doi: 10.1007/s11136-021-03063-1. Epub 2022 Jan 24. PMID: 35072904; PMCID: PMC8785005.

Mental Capacity Act (2005). Department of Health. London: The Stationary Office.

Mental Health Act (1983) (amended 2007). Department of Health. London: The Stationary Office.

National Collaborating Centre for Mental Health (2021). The community mental health framework for adults and older adults: support, care and treatment. www.rcpsych.ac.uk/docs/default-source/improving-care/nccmh/the-community-mental-health-framework-for-adults-and-older-adults-full-guidance/part-1-the-community-mental-health-framework-for-adults-and-older-adults---support-care-and-treatment---nccmh---march-2021.pdf [Accessed 27th November 2024].

NHS Digital (2024). Mental Health Bulletin, 2023-24 annual report. https://digital.nhs.uk/data-and-information/publications/statistical/mental-health-bulletin/2023-24-annual-report [Accessed 27th November 2024].

NHS England (2024). Getting a assessment. www.nhs.uk/conditions/social-care-and-support-guide/help-from-social-services-and-charities/getting-a-needs-assessment/ [14th November 2024].

NHS England (2024). Guidance to integrated care boards on intensive and assertive community mental health care. www.england.nhs.uk/long-read/guidance-to-integrated-care-boards-on-intensive-and-assertive-community-mental-health-care/ [Accessed 2nd November 2024].

NHS England (2023). Mental health of Children and Young People in England, 2023 – wave 4 follow up to the 2017 survey. https://digital.nhs.uk/data-and-information/publications/statistical/mental-health-of-children-and-young-people-in-england/2023-wave-4-follow-up [Accessed 28th November 2024].

NHS England (2023). Supported self-management: peer support guide. www.england.nhs.uk/long-read/peer-support/ [Accessed 28th November 2024].

NHS England (2022). Care programme approach. www.england.nhs.uk/wp-content/uploads/2021/07/B0526-care-programme-approach-position-statement-v2.pdf [Accessed 21st November 2024].

NHS England (2022). Integrated care systems: what are they and case studies. www.england.nhs.uk/integratedcare/

NHS England (2019). NHS long term plan. [Accessed 1st November 2024].

NHS England (2019). NHS Mental Health Implementation Plan. www.longtermplan.nhs.uk/wp-content/uploads/2019/07/nhs-mental-health-implementation-plan-2019-20-2023-24.pdf [Accessed 28th November 2024].

NHS England (2016). Adult Psychiatry Morbidity Survey: Survey of Mental Health and Wellbeing, England, 2014. https://digital.nhs.uk/data-and-information/publications/statistical/adult-psychiatric-morbidity-survey/adult-psychiatric-morbidity-survey-survey-of-mental-health-and-wellbeing-england-2014 [Accessed 12th November 2024].

Nuffield Trust (2024). Follow-up care for people discharged from mental health inpatient care. www.nuffieldtrust.org.uk/resource/follow-up-care-for-adults-with-mental-health-problems [Accessed 8th November 2024].

Priebe, S., McCabe, R., and Bullenkamp, J. (2007). Structured patient-clinician communication and one-year outcome in community mental health care: a cluster randomised controlled trial. *British Journal of Psychiatry* 191: 420–426. doi: 10.1192/bjp.bp.107.036939

PSR (n.d.). The Priority Services Register. www.thepsr.co.uk/#about-psr [Accessed 15th November 2024].

Royal College of Psychiatrists (2021). Social prescribing. www.rcpsych.ac.uk/mental-health/treatments-and-wellbeing/social-prescribing#:~:text=Social%20prescribing%20helps%20to%20connect%20people%20with%20mental%20or%20physical,medication%20involved%20in%20social%20prescribing [Accessed 11th November 2024].

Royal College of Psychiatrists (2017). Good psychiatric practice. Confidentiality and information sharing. Third edition. www.rcpsych.ac.uk/docs/default-source/improving-care/better-mh-policy/college-reports/college-report-cr209.pdf?sfvrsn=23858153_2 [Accessed 4th November 2024].

Sanders, R. (2020). ESSS Outline. Carers mental and physical health. www.iriss.org.uk/sites/default/files/2020-10/esss_outline_carers_mental_physical_health.pdf [Accessed 9th November 2024].

Smith, F. (2024). Money and Mental Health Policy Institute. Reforming the Mental Health Ct. Time to tackle the links between financial difficulty and acute mental illness. www.moneyandmentalhealth.org/wp-content/uploads/2024/10/Reforming-the-Mental-Health-Act.pdf [Accessed 21st November 2024].

Sugarman, D. E. (2023). Telemental health for clinical assessment and treatment. *British Medical Journal.* 380. doi: 10.1136/bmj-2022-072398

The Carers Trust (2023). The triangle of care: carers included. A guide to best practice in health care. https://carers.org/downloads/triangle-of-care-a4-2pp-leaflet-(health-care)-web-pink.pdf [Accessed 12th November 2024].

The King's Fund (October 2024) Response to care quality commission report. www.kingsfund.org.uk/insight-and-analysis/press-releases/response-annual-CQC-state-care-report-2024.

The King's Fund (August 2022). Integrated care systems explained (2022 August). www.kingsfund.org.uk/insight-and-analysis/long-reads/integrated-care-systems-explained

The King's Fund (2020). Briefing. www.kingsfund.org.uk/insight-and-analysis/reports/mental-health-primary-care-networks

The King's Fund (2015). Briefing. https://assets.kingsfund.org.uk/f/256914/x/78db101b90/mental_health_under_pressure_2015.pdf [Accessed 28th November 2024].

Turner, J., Hayward, R., Angel, K., Fulford, B., Hall, J., and Millard, C., Thomson, M. (2015). The history of mental health services in modern England: practitioner memories and the direction of future research. *Medicine History* 59(4): 599–624. doi: 10.1017/mdh.2015.48. PMID: 26352306; PMCID: PMC4595954.

UNICEF (2021). Closing the digital divide for good. *Executive Summary.* www.unicef.org.uk/wp-content/uploads/2021/06/Closing-the-Digital-Divide-for-Good_ExecSum.pdf [Accessed 13th January 2025].

Wade, D. T., and Halligan, P. W. (2017). The biopsychosocial model of illness: a model whose time has come. *Clinical Rehabilitation.* 31(8): 995–1004.

7 Compulsory Admission into Hospital (Restricted and Non-restricted)

Ahmad F Ramjhun

Introduction

It is important to acknowledge from the outset that compulsory admissions to hospital do not sit at all well with human rights and directly conflict with Article 8 of the European Convention on Human Rights, (1951), (ECHR), considering a person's right to privacy, respect, and family life. It is therefore no coincidence that this conflict has captured minds and continues to cause controversy. The Independent Review of the Mental Health Act, (2018), (IRMHA), (Department of Health and Social Care, 2018), reflects and echoes this tension- as it juxtaposes the rights of individuals versus the preservation of life and the protection of others (Kelly, 2016). Compulsory detention only arises from extreme circumstances where hospital is the only resort. Many patients have mental disorders which are chronic, relapsing and remitting in nature, reaching a degree where their symptoms are causing serious distress and concerns, presenting with high risks to themselves and others such as self-harming, suicide attempts, dangerous and/or sometimes criminal behaviours. Most suffer from schizophrenia, psychosis, affective disorders, and personality disorders, including some with treatment-resistant disorders, often compounded with alcohol and/or substance misuse. There are times when preservation of life is paramount, when detention is unquestionably the only lawful decision; for example, where the risks of suicide, extreme starvation through food refusal or fatal self-injuries are very high or where other people are in serious danger. Where a person or the public is at risk of serious harm and injury, the right to life has to take precedence against all others. The risk must be serious and the degree of danger high, greatly exceeding the need for general safety in order to meet the statutory threshold envisaged in CoP, (Department of Health and Social Care, 2018).

Patients are not only detained in hospital solely for their health and/or safety and/or for the protection of others. This, alone, is not lawful; there must also be assessment and/or the availability of appropriate medical treatment, (IRMHA, 2018). There must be an assessment provided and a therapeutic intervention that addresses the mental disorder, even if this only serves to alleviate or prevent its worsening or one or more of its symptoms, Mental Health Act 1983 (MHA 1983) (Section S)145(4). Therapeutic intervention is broadly defined. It is not restricted to medical treatment alone, going well beyond this, to include for example, nursing care, occupational therapy, and psychology within a holistic therapeutic regime (S145(1)).

Detentions also have to be the least restrictive available option as enshrined in law. If a person can be supported in an environment other than hospital then this must be considered. In some cases a Deprivation of Liberty Safeguard (DoLS) could be considered using the Mental Capacity Act 2005, (MCA) – as amended in 2019. For example, in *ML -v- (1) Priory Healthcare Limited) [2023] SSJ [2023] UKUT 237 (AAC)*, which was an Upper Tribunal appeal against a decision of a Mental Health Review Tribunal (MHRT). In this judgement it was held that

DOI: 10.4324/9781003635543-8

detention of a high-risk patient serving a life term for murder arising from diminished responsibility was unlawful. This was because the tribunal failed to consider the least restrictive option in that the use of Deprivation of Liberty Safeguards would have enabled him to be discharged, given that the main requirement was for him to comply with medication and that his risks were no longer at a level to justify continued detention. Similarly, in *SS v Cornwall Partnership NHS Foundation Trust (Mental Health) [2023] UKUT 258 (AAC)*, it was also found that discharge into the community was a realistic alternative to detention in hospital if suitable aftercare was available.

In terms of the numbers of people who are compulsorily detained, the data from NHS England Mental Health Act Statistics (NHS MHA Stat), (2023), shows that as of October 2022, there were 53,337 new detentions in hospital. This was, of course, towards the tail end of the Covid-19 pandemic, and has been increasing since 2018, i.e., before the pandemic. In 2018–19 it totalled 49, 988, increasing to 50,989 in 2019-20 at the start of the pandemic, (NHS MHA Stat 2019, 2020). The 2021-22 data is thought to be an under-estimate, due to inconsistency of reporting and the incompleteness of data. Detention rates were higher for males, (93.8 per 100,000) than females (86.4 per 100,000). They tend to decline with age, with the highest detention rates amongst the 18-34 age group, being 67% higher than amongst those aged 65 plus. Black, Ethnic, and Minority Ethnic groups were between 4 to 11 times over-represented when compared with the general population.

In terms of restricted patients, a total of 1,746 restricted patients were admitted (new admissions and recalls), not vastly changed since 2008, with a 5% increase from 2022. Of the total population of restricted patients about 65% were White, 18% Black and 8% Asian, showing little change from the previous year. A total of 73 (4%) of admissions were into high secure hospitals. As the figures above shows, the over-representation of Black, Ethnic, and Minority Ethnic groups in detention has been known for some time, (Barnett et al., 2019; MHA Statistics 2023), and remains a continuing concern (IRMHA, 2018). They have an increased risk of involuntary psychiatric care, continuing to experience "profound inequalities" with regard to their access to care and treatment, (IRMHA, (b) 1998, p.7). Amongst these, black African and Caribbean men constitute the highest numbers detained at 11 times the general population. The reasons are far from clear and may be due to a multiplicity of factors, ranging from poverty, deprivation, discrimination, and social disadvantage; compounded by structural factors linked with fear, intolerance, stigma, stereotyping, and racism (IRMHA, 2018).

Tribunals and Compulsory Detentions

The MHA 1983 makes a number of provisions for detention in hospitals; this chapter focuses only on the main sections. The MHA 1983 defines "mental disorder" as any disorder or disability of the mind. Dependence on alcohol or drugs is not, [(S1(3)], unless the impact of any such dependency and how this relates to the mental disorder can be shown. Learning Disability (LD) means an arrested or incomplete development of the mind which includes significant impairment of intelligence and social functioning (S1(4). However, an LD alone does not amount to or constitute a mental disorder unless it is also associated with **Abnormally Aggressive or Seriously Irresponsible Conduct [S 1(4) and 1(2a)]**. It is noteworthy that neither Abnormally Aggressive nor Seriously Irresponsible Conduct are defined in the MHA 1983 though they are determinative.

Abnormally Aggressive behaviour is not simply being aggressive but must reach the higher threshold and levels of abnormality required by law. This may sometimes be self-evident.

However, it should always be considered in terms of its disproportionality; its frequency, intensity and severity, duration and persistence and the extent to which this gives rise to serious risks to the health and safety of the person and others (CoP; Department of Health, 2015).

In regard to Seriously Irresponsible Conduct, caselaw has clarified the position on what constitutes Seriously Irresponsible Conduct. In F (Mental Health Act: Guardianship) (2000) [1 FLR 192] the Court favoured a narrow and restrictive interpretation in the case of a patient with LD seeking to return home to possible abuse where there were also known and longstanding issues of neglect and inadequate parenting. It found that this was not seriously irresponsible. The Court in Newham LBC v S (2003) [EWHC 1909 Fam] also held that a lack of road sense and a tendency to rush into the road without looking did not, in the circumstances of that case, constitute seriously irresponsible behaviour for the purpose of mental disorder. However, in GC vs Managers of the Kingswood Centre et al (2008) [7784/2008]; the Court arrived at a different view. This dealt with a person suffering with a compulsion to pick up litter even on the road. He had been knocked down before but still persisted, not considering himself vulnerable. The Court held that a tendency to rush onto the road could not be argued to be always not seriously irresponsible. Each case therefore very much turns on its own facts. What is also clear is that guardianship is most unlikely for those with an LD unless they also have a mental disorder, i.e., in that they also present with abnormally aggressive or seriously irresponsible conduct.

Responsible Clinician (RC)

Responsible Clinicians used to be psychiatrists; however this role was extended to other mental health professionals such as experienced psychologists and nurses in the 2007 amendments to the MHA (1983). This was to facilitate the use of a wider professional workforce and set of skills, best suited to deliver an enhanced service to the patient. The RC is the clinician approved by the Secretary of State or other body with authority to exercise such powers on their behalf. Effectively they have overall responsibility for patients.

Approved Mental Health Practitioner (AMHP)

The AMHP is tasked with considering the medical recommendations and can then decide on whether or not it is necessary to make an application for detention under S2. If in agreement, they have the power to arrange and enforce detention, usually through the ambulance or the police.

Nearest Relative

Section 26 of the MHA, (1983) sets out who is the Nearest Relative (NR) for anyone kept in hospital under Sections 2, 3,4 or 37, on a CTO or under a guardianship. This might be a spouse, parent, adoptive relative- though not a step relative- or sibling, and is not the same as the next of kin who does not have any rights under the MHA. The NR is normally someone whom the patient trusts. It represents an important safeguard though this might be subject to review, given that the IRMHA (2018) considers that it is outdated, proposing the concept of a Nominated Person (NP) who can be chosen. A Nearest Relative can make an application for detention under Section 2 or 3 or ask the hospital managers for discharge. In relation to discharge, this can only be resisted through a Barring Order issued by the Responsible Clinician (RC) (Barber et al., 2012).

Admission for Assessment – Section 2

An admission under Section 2 (S2) for assessment may be made on the grounds that a patient is suffering from mental disorder of a nature or degree which warrants their detention in a hospital for assessment (or for assessment followed by medical treatment) for at least a limited period of up to 28 days, in the interests of the patient's own health or safety or that of others. If at the end of this period, further detention is considered appropriate, an assessment for Section 3 would need to be carried out. A S2 admission is usually based on the written recommendations of two registered medical practitioners, confirming that the legal criteria are met. One of these should have previous acquaintance with the patient, if practicable. The threshold is low in this regard in that previous personal acquaintance is not necessary; it only requires the doctor not to be dealing with the patient's case in an uninformed or unprepared way (*Reed (Trainer v Bronglais Hospital et al.) (2001)*)[EWHC 792 Admin]. A court in the case, *TTM v Hackney 2011 [EWCA, Civ 4]* also held that even if this condition was not met, this would not invalidate the Section, finding that even the briefest of contact or some knowledge from reading of medical notes was sufficient.

The MHA Code of Practice, (Department of Health, 2015) was therefore suitably amended to reflect this judgement, lending way to a pragmatic approach, emphasising the issue of practicability.

Admission for Treatment – Section 3

An application for admission for treatment may be made in respect of a patient on the grounds that they are suffering from mental disorder of **a nature or degree** requiring them to receive medical treatment available in a hospital for their health or safety or for the protection of others. This can be for up to six months and if further treatment is necessary, can be renewed initially for a further six months, and thereafter for periods of 12 months. S3 detention often follows S2 where a patient initially admitted under S2 requires further assessment and treatment, e.g., where the assessment is incomplete or where the treatment needs to be consolidated, particularly where the medication used requires titration. Patients on S3 can be placed on Community Treatment Orders (CTOs) (see below) and discharged home, under a number of conditions, if it is deemed that their treatment could continue in the community.

Community Treatment Order (CTO)

A CTO can be used for people detained in hospital for treatment (Section 3 or 37 Notional (N)) where the responsible clinician (RC) considers that this treatment does not need to be in hospital and can be in the community, but that they are unlikely to comply in the absence of a CTO and that the power of recall is necessary. CTOs come with conditions to promote the person's ongoing treatment and recovery. Failure to comply with these can result in them being recalled to and re-detained in hospital. CTOs were initially introduced in 2007 and can only be made if the AMHP agrees. They are intended to avoid inappropriate or extended S17 leave; in these cases, the RC must consider a CTO if this is for more than seven days. Their efficacy is in question; Burns et al., (2013), considered them to be largely ineffective. There is also concern that they are overused with an increasing call for them to be dramatically reduced (IMRMHA, op cit.). They may well be abandoned in the future if the situation does not change. Indeed, the IMRMHA even goes on so far as to say that: "CTOs are in the 'Last Chance Saloon'", (IRMHA, 2018, p. 15).

Emergency Admission – Section 4

In an emergency situation a person can be detained for up to 72 hours based on only one medical recommendation, and an AMHP application, during which time another doctor may complete the second recommendation necessary for a Section 2.

Discharge

The RC in overall charge of the patient's assessment or treatment may discharge the patient from detention at any time.

Standard of Proof

In tribunals, the standard of proof is always the civil standard, on a balance of probabilities test, i.e. 'more likely than not' *(R (AN) v MHRT (Northern Region) (2005) [EWCA Civ 1605]*. The burden is on the Responsible Authority. Previously this was on the patient but it was reversed due to its incompatibility with the Human Rights Act 1998 (Barber et al op.cit.).

There is only one exception, which is where a patient who is subject to Section 41 applies for an absolute discharge, where the burden is on the patient, see *RH v South London and Maudsley NHS Foundation Trust, (2010) [EWCA civ 1273]*.

Patients with Criminal Convictions and Awaiting Sentence

These patients differ from those described earlier, in that they either have a criminal conviction or they are awaiting sentence, dependent on which Section they are subject to. Broadly speaking, they are those for whom it has been decided that they should be admitted to hospital for treatment, rather than prison.

Section 37 (Hospital Order)

This can be imposed by a Criminal Court on the basis of two medical recommendations, with one of the doctors having given evidence orally.

Section 41 (Restriction Order)

Section 37 can be combined with Section 41 (Restriction Order) MHA when it is necessary to protect the public from serious harm rather than just the risk of further offending. This restriction prevents the offender from leaving hospital either on leave or discharge or from transferring to a different hospital. The Secretary of State who retains overall responsibility must consent to this, bearing in mind the risk to the public. In *R v Birch (1990) Court of Appeal [CR App R 78]* it was held that the risk to the public must be there. That risk was not found in a patient under Section 37/41; Section 41 was therefore quashed, with the patient remaining under Section 37. Where a prisoner transferred from prison for treatment in hospital under Section 47 (hospital transfer) has served their sentence and their release date has passed, they become a notional Section 37 patient (S37N); i.e. restrictions no longer apply in the same way and they are treated as if they are under S37.

A hospital order cannot be made where the sentence is fixed by law – for example in cases of murder which carry a mandatory life sentence (S37; Parole Board 2020). The Secretary of State can, however, make a direction under Section 47 for a transfer to hospital rather than prison on the same day that a court sentences the offender.

Sections 45A, 47, 48 and 49: transfer of prisoners.

S45A is sometimes referred to as a hybrid order because of its dual nature in combining a hospital and a limitation direction. The hospital direction has the same force as a transfer direction to hospital under S47 whilst the limitation direction has the same effect as the restriction imposed under S49.

S47 is for treatment of prisoners in hospital but will usually have S49 attached, unless the patient is nearing the end of their sentence. S49 is a restriction order with the same restrictions as those that apply under S41.

S48 is for the transfer to hospital for urgent treatment of unsentenced prisoners and others in remand and immigration detention centres. This is known as a transfer direction and is for people still facing on-going proceedings in Court; it ceases to have effect when these are concluded.

Any discharge of restricted patients under S45A and 47/49 must be approved by the Secretary of State. This means a discharge from hospital only and does not exclude consideration of a return back to prison (R *(on the application of Abu Rideh) v MHRT (2004)* [EWHC 1999 Admin].

The MHRT can consider whether a patient is entitled to be conditionally or absolutely discharged and will apply the S73 criteria.

The Criteria to be Considered – Nature, Degree, Risk and Appropriate Medical Treatment

Nature – this is the type of mental disorder, its diagnosis and clinical features, such as its duration, its regularity, re-occurrence or chronicity, and whether it is constant, relapsing, remitting, and responsive to treatment, in addition to issues such as risk-related behaviour (*see also R v Mental Health Review Tribunal for the South Thames Region ex parte Smith 1999 [COD 948]; CoP 14.6*). Nature may be sufficient on its own to make detention appropriate even if the degree in the particular case does not. Another consideration is whether the disorder would relapse in the absence of medication. Whilst it was previously held that the probability of risk in the community must be in the near future [(*R (Moyle) v London South and South West Region MHRT (1999)*) [MHLR 195]; *CH v Derbyshire Healthcare NHS FT (2011) UKUT 129 [AAC]*, this is no longer the case.

In LW v Cornwall Partnership NHS Foundation Trust [2018] UKUT 408 [AAC], it was accepted that in cases where there is a risk of a relapse, how soon that is likely to occur is relevant but that the risks to self and/or others are also significant. The court concluded that any likely relapse need not be "soon", "in the near future" or within the permitted duration of a CTO or for any S3 detention.

Degree – refers to the current manifestations or symptoms of the mental disorder, such as hallucinations, delusional convictions, and beliefs or paranoia (*R v Mental Health Review Tribunal for the South Thames Region ex parte Smith (1999) [COD 948]*). Degree can include the level and/or absence of insight; the presenting symptoms; the levels of distressing and incapacitating thoughts; fixations, suicidal ideations, anxieties, and commands that the person feels compelled to act on; their emotions and levels of distress. The way they communicate and behave are also important and can often be self-evident, e.g., pressure of speech; tangential thinking, flight of ideas; disjointed communication, lacking focus, with irrelevancies and difficult to interrupt. Behaviours such as self-harming, aggression and/or threats and danger to others are, of course, obvious. These manifestations or symptoms will help assess the severity of the disorder. A tribunal will be considering how severe this is at the time of the hearing and not necessarily how it was before. It will also consider degree separately to nature. In some cases, the nature of the disorder may be that the patient can normally be managed in the community, but the current manifestation prevents that and either warrants detention for assessment or makes detention appropriate for treatment.

Risks – must be serious and be linked to the mental disorder, affecting health either mental or physical, including the likelihood of relapse. They also include safety risks in terms of self-harm, dangerous and reckless behaviour, suicide and vulnerability to exploitation and harm. The protection of others is also key in relation to any possible acts of aggression and violence, including arson- whether pre-meditated or accidental- and psychological harm. Dangerous driving, jumping from bridges or onto railway lines - sometimes forming part of planned suicide attempts - also carry serious risks to others. Again, it is worth highlighting that the three different risk aspects are considered individually by the tribunal, *risk to the person's health, their safety, and the protection of others.*

Appropriate Medical Treatment – must be actually available, (CoP, op cit. p 248). This is not the same as the previous "treatability test" under the previous legislation now removed, i.e., before the MHA 1983 was amended (Barber et al., 2012). Whilst the treatability test is whether the disorder is amenable to treatment, the availability test focuses on whether that treatment is available in the particular hospital concerned. The disorder might also be treatable, but the treatment proposed by the Responsible Authority (RA) may not be the appropriate treatment and this must remain as a key factor. This is nevertheless a lower threshold than treatability. In *MD v Nottingham Healthcare NHS Trust, (2010) UKUT 59[AAC]*, it was held that the provision of a structured and protective setting on a ward, not only reduces risks but can also amount to appropriate medical treatment if this helped to alleviate or prevent the worsening of symptoms. This is, of course, not an immediate solution and until the treatment takes its course, the patient or others may suffer. *SF v Avon and Wiltshire Mental Health Partnership NHS Trust and RB, (2023), UKUT (2005) [AAC]* clarified the position further in this regard. This was a case of a severely ill and neuro-diverse patient who needed psychology and psycho-social support not available on an acute ward. All parties agreed the environment was not beneficial and likely to be non-therapeutic and counter-productive, albeit that the risks were being managed and she was being kept safe. It was held that medical treatment was not available in this case. Although the nature, safety, and risk criteria were satisfied, the latter was not. The judge found that medical treatment may not be appropriate or available if it is not tailored to the patient's diagnosis. Essential treatment in this case-psychology-was not available.

It is clear that detention can only be lawful if the legal criteria are met. The MHA 1983 talks about either nature *or* degree and likewise differentiates between the 3 limbs of the risk criteria in terms of health *or* safety *or* safety of others whilst using the word *and* for medical treatment. The availability and appropriateness of medical treatment was determinative here in that it is pointless to detain a patient in a hospital when this serves no medical purpose and when indeed, this was making the patient worse, not better. Therefore, the test with regard to medical treatment was not met.

Appeals Against Detention

Appeals against S2 detentions can be made by patients or referrals made by the Secretary of State (SoS). These can only be done once during the 14-day period starting on the day of admission. For those already in hospital informally, this is the date when the formal Section 2 started.

The Nearest Relative can apply and Hospital Managers (HM) or the Secretary of State (SoS) may also make a referral, but this is restricted to S3 only. Detention under S2 is most often used with patients with first onset psychosis or mood disorder or those who require a first and/or further assessment of their disorder in a hospital due to a significant change in presentation. Some would be re-admissions due to relapse. They often present with acute, distressing, and life-threatening risks; many with acute thought and/or eating disorders, mood changes, self-harming, and suicidal ideation. Most suffer from schizophrenia and other psychotic or affective disorders- all with high degree of risks in terms of their health and/or safety, and/or that of others. Many respond to treatment and are discharged without the need for a tribunal appeal; some voluntarily remain in hospital informally.

Appeals for Absolute Discharge

Where a restricted patient is seeking absolute discharge, the key issues relate to the nature and gravity of the index offence and the risks this may continue to pose in addition to the nature and degree of the mental disorder, including its history and trajectory. Whether the power of recall remains appropriate will also be amongst the key considerations, with the focus on health and safety and the prevention of harm to both the patient and the public.

R (SC) v MHRT (2005) [EWHC 17 Admin] was a judicial review application of a conditionally discharged restricted patient seeking an absolute discharge. Amongst the claims, it was argued that the MHA 1983 provided no criteria whatsoever in relation to his Section 75(2) application only stating those that do not apply. In dismissing the case, the Court detailed the criteria applicable in such cases.

These are summarised below and provide guidance in terms of applications for absolute discharge. Tribunals will consider:

- The index offence; its nature, seriousness and gravity, and the circumstances in which this took place e.g., manslaughter through diminished responsibility, arson; serious harm to others or to self; the context, background and any triggers and relevant circumstantial factors.
- The current disorder; its nature, degree, and gravity, including any history in terms of its chronicity, any past re-occurrences and relapses and any likely risks in the future.
- The risk and likelihood of the patient re-offending and the degree of harm the public would be exposed to if they were to re-offend.
- The risk and likelihood of the patient needing to be recalled in the future for further treatment in hospital, e.g., due to relapse; risky behaviours or non-compliance with treatment.
- The nature of any conditions previously imposed; why these were necessary and the extent to which they should either continue or be changed in any way.

S v Elysium Healthcare & Secretary of State for Justice (2021) UKUT186 [AAC]; makes clear that restricted patients must not be dealt with more severely than anyone else.

Dilemmas in Decision Making

Patients with severe anorexia, those planning to jump on the railway line or from bridges; others setting fire to their flats or waving a weapon in public intent on attacking others – in the erroneous belief that this is what they must do either because of voices ordering them to do so or because they have become extremely paranoid and think they must defend themselves – are common cases where decision making is obvious. It is so difficult to imagine how they must feel being driven to such acts of desperation, losing self-control. Common sense says that removal to receive assessment, care or treatment is necessary and the law – whether under Section (S) 2 or Section 3 of the Mental Health Act, (MHA), 1983 – allows for compulsory admission. This is straightforward. Nevertheless, amidst all this upheaval and stresses, it is crucial to maintain a humane approach, not losing sight of their suffering, their extreme distress, and the impact on their families. These are critical times never to be underestimated. There are also other cases where detention needs to be subject to greater scrutiny. This is where there is little or no risk to self or others, and the whole rationale is based on the nature and not the degree of the disorder. I have experience of dealing with cases of patients with treatment resistant schizophrenia with their main issues being non-compliance with medication, which has caused bizarre behaviours and self-neglect. Some as a result were living in poor and nearly uninhabitable accommodation. These persons have been living in the community for years albeit with a quality of life that is perceived to be less than ideal and continue to have a remitting, relapsing disorder with crises, giving rise to concerns from professionals, neighbours, or relatives. There is no actual physical harm to anyone. There are also others detained because their behaviours are unusual, perhaps perceived to have unusual and extreme beliefs, such as being watched or controlled by the television or openly expressing and practising their religious beliefs, including those who believe they are God or being commanded to act in a certain way. The question is how far these perceptions or so-called psychotic symptoms matter and the extent to which these critically impact on the patient's capabilities and ability to function. This is never easy; with professionals facing agonising, and critical decisions. The crucial task in these types of presentation is being able to identify the nature, degree, and risks that the disorder presents with, if any, and if indeed there is a mental disorder. The statutory criteria must always be satisfied. The "Winterwerp" criteria (1979) make it clear that there must be reliable and objective medical evidence to show that the person is of unsound mind and suffering from a "true" mental disorder (*Winterwerp v The Netherlands Judgment, 1979;* p.15), of a nature or degree to justify detention. This is much more and very different from them simply behaving or having beliefs perceived to be deviant from norms in society (*R v Mental Health Review Tribunal for the South Thames Region ex parte Smith [1999] COD 948*).

Patients' Experiences

It is worth acknowledging the obvious point that detention is a last resort, should only be used when the risks a person presents to their own health and/or safety and/or the safety of others are so high that they could not be treated or managed without compulsion or in a less restrictive environment such as in the community, or informally. It is always a difficult and extreme decision to make, and any action must be compliant with the law, with particular regard to the MHA statutory criteria. It is safe to assume that no one would ever wish to have their freedom, dignity, and autonomy removed in this way, especially at a time when they are at their most vulnerable and in crisis. If this is the only way to help and keep them and/or others safe, then they must be treated with care, respect, compassion, and dignity. Behind any detained patient is a person, full of fear, often very confused with little insight or understanding, but facing loss of control over their lives (see the Independent Review of the Mental Health Act – IRMHA) (Modernising the Mental Health Act, 2018). It is no wonder that they may be presenting at their worst and most vulnerable, in crisis. They must continue to have a voice and, even when so unwell, need to be actively listened to. This is where any advanced decisions they may have made, (see IRMHA, 2018) may assist. Patients so detained report losing their freedom and dignity and becoming distressed, fearful, and wary of authority, (IRMHA, 2018; Fenton et al., 2014). Detention does not ease their pain, their mistrusts and their anxieties nor do they necessarily see this intrusion into their privacy and into their lives as protection, especially when there has been no wrong-doing, (Chambers et al., 2014).

Looking to the Future

It is difficult to predict or second guess the legislative changes or reforms that are likely to arise from the recommendations of IRMHA (2018). These have been on the table for some time, and it is difficult to say how much or how little of these, if any, will be enacted. Whilst the changes suggested are not ground-breaking, there is so much to commend in terms of increasing choice and reducing compulsion, not least the focus on the IRMHA's four core principles of:

1. *Choice and Autonomy*- e.g. increased involvement in decision making; advance decisions; greater legal safeguards with regard to Electro-Convulsive Therapy (ECT); right to advocacy; powers of attorney as in the Mental Capacity Act 2005 as amended in 2019, and the moving away from Nearest Relative to the Nominated Person.
2. *Least Restriction*- least invasive and least restrictive intervention; and lesser coercion including a shift from compulsion to more rights-based approaches.
3. *Therapeutic Benefit*- central and core to detention; availability and appropriateness of treatment; ceasing the use of police cells and finding more therapeutic alternatives and safe places not those which have previously caused or elicited trauma; statutory care plans that can focus on recovery and be informed by the patient's views and advance choices which are amenable to evaluation as to the therapeutic goals and outcomes.
4. *Person as an individual*- greater use of holistic, person-centred approaches focusing on recovery as a process, not a cure which may not be an attainable destination.

   For example, the Recovery Model which has been gaining momentum is useful. This moves away from pathology, goes beyond elimination of symptoms, and focuses on wellness, and well-being to move towards social recovery. It is patient directed; a process, a journey, not a single event or a destination (Mountain and Shah 2008; Department of Health 2001; Expert Group on Mental Health Policy 2006). This should work alongside appropriate medical treatment.

None of these are novel and/or contentious; the proposed powers for tribunals to challenge treatment is perhaps new. The comments against each of the core principles are mine and not necessarily consistent or dealt in the same order as the IMHAR, (2018). Nevertheless, whilst none is surprising, the question is why they arose and are the cause of such concerns.

Conclusion

We clearly have a long way to go if we are to further improve the quality of life and the experiences of those detained. Mental health services are under enormous pressure, and they do make a huge difference, not least in saving lives, providing quality treatment, and reducing risks. There is no doubt about this. Service and resource pressures in addition to the shortage of available beds, however, inevitably impact on service delivery. We are fortunate in the UK to have a tried and tested system that has provided excellent quality care, treatment, and safety for our most vulnerable citizens; the dedication and commitment of staff, working in difficult and challenging circumstances is without doubt. There are some difficulties and issues mainly due to lack of staff and resources. Very rarely there are some serious issues uncovered as with

Winterbourne, (Department of Health, 2012), but they are hopefully outliers, outside the norm and should not cloud perceptions of service improvements made over the years. Mental health is not alone in terms of needing to continually improve and modernise. However, modernisation will not be achieved by strategies and increased service provision alone. It requires greater transparency within a culture of trust and mutual self-respect, (IRMHA, 2018). It will perform *even* better with greater scrutiny; more self-questioning and more in-depth analysis and evaluation of what works. Time will tell if the modernisation needed happens.

Acknowledgment

My thanks to Tribunal Judges Mostyn Evans and Katherine Gibson for kindly reading and commenting on my draft.

Bibliography

Barber P, Brown R, Martin D (2012) *Mental Health Law in England and Wales.* Sage.

Barnett P, Mackay E, Matthews H, Gate R, Greenwood H, Ariyo K, Bhui K, Halvorsrud K, Pilling, Smith S (2019) Ethnic variations in compulsory detention under the Mental Health Act: a systematic review and meta-analysis of international data. *Lancet Psychiatry.* **6**: 305–17.

Burns T, Rugkasa J, Molodynski A et al (2013) Community treatment orders for patients with psychosis (OCTET): a randomised controlled trial. *Lancet.* **3821**: 1627–33.

Chambers M, Gallagher A, Borschmann R, Gillard S, Turner K, Kantaris X (2014) The experiences of detained mental health service users: issues of dignity in care. *BMC Medical Ethics.* **15**: 8–19.

Department of Health (2001) *The Journey to Recovery: The Government's Vision for Mental Health Care.* Department of Health.

Department of Health (2012) *Transforming care: A national response to Winterbourne View Hospital: Department of Health Review Final Report.* Department of Health.

Department of Health (2015) *Mental Health Act 1983: Code of Practice.* Stationery Office.

Department of Health and Social Care (2018) Modernising the Mental Health Act - final report from the independent review IRMHA. Online Modernising the Mental Health Act – final report from the independent review - GOV.UK

Expert Group on Mental Health Policy (2006) *A Vision for Change: Report of the Expert Group on Mental Health Policy.* Stationery Office.

Fenton K, Larkin M, Boden ZVR, Thompson J, Hickman G, Newton E (2014) The experiential impact of hospitalisation in early psychosis: service-user accounts of inpatient environments. *Health Place.* **30**: 234–41.

Jacobson N, Greenley D (2001) What is recovery? A conceptual model and explication. *Psychiatric Services.* **52**: 482–5.

Kelly B (2016) *Mental Illness, Human Rights and the Law (2016).* Royal College of Psychiatrists.

Mental Capacity Act (2005) www.Legislation.gov.uk

Ministry of Justice (2023) *Restricted Patients Statistics: 2023 England and Wales: 25 April 2024.* Crown.

Modernising the Mental Health Act (2018) *Increasing Choice, Reducing Compulsion: Final Report of the Independent Review of the Mental Health Act 1983.* Crown.

Modernising the Mental Health Act (2018 (a)) *Increasing Choice, Reducing Compulsion Final Report of the Independent Review of the Mental Health Act 1983- Summary Version.* London Stationary Office

Mountain D, Shah P (2008) Recovery and the medical model. *Advances in Psychiatric Treatment.* **14**: 241–244. doi: 10.1192/apt.bp.107.004671

NHS Digital (2019) Mental Health Act Statistics *Annual Figures 2018-19: 29 October 2019.* https://digital.nhs.uk/data-and-information/publications/statistical/mental-health-act-statistics-annual-figures/2019-20-annual-figures

NHS Digital (2020) Mental Health Act Statistics *Annual Figures 2019-20: 27 October 2020.* https://digi
tal.nhs.uk/data-and-information/publications/statistical/mental-health-act-statistics-annual-figures/
2019-20-annual-figures

NHS Digital (2022) Mental Health Act Statistics *Annual Figures 2021-22: 27 October2022.* https://digital.
nhs.uk/data-and-information/publications/statistical/health-survey-for-england/2022-part-2

The Parole Board (2020) Guidance on Restricted Patients and the Mental Health Act October 2020 **v1.0**
Gov.uk.

Caselaw

CH v Derbyshire Healthcare NHS FT [2011] UKUT 129 AAC

F (Mental Health Act: Guardianship) [20020] 1 FLR 192)

LW v Cornwall Partnership NHS Foundation Trust [2018] UKUT 408 (AAC)

MD v Nottingham Healthcare NHS Trust (2010) UKUT 59 (AAC)

ML -v- (1) Priory Healthcare Limited and (2) SSJ [2023] UKUT 237 (AAC)

Newham LBC v BS [2003] EWHC 1909 (Fam)

R v Birch (1990) Court of Appeal [CR App R 78]

R (on the application of Abu Rideh) v MHRT [2004] EWHC 1999 (Admin)

R (AN) v MHRT (Northern Region) [2005] EWCA Civ 1605)

R(GC) vs Managers of the Kingswood Centre of Central and North West London NHS Foundation Trust.
(CO/7784/2008)

R (Moyle) v London South and South West Region MHRT [1999] MHLR 195

R v Mental Health Review Tribunal for the South Thames Region ex parte Smith [1999] COD 948

R v MHRT, ex p Hall [1999] EWHC Admin 351

R (SC) v MHRT [2005] EWHC 17 (Admin).

R (Smith) v MHRT South Thames Region [1998] EWHC Admin 832

RB v Nottinghamshire Healthcare NHS Trust [2011] UKUT 73 (AAC)

Reed (Trainer) v Bronglais Hospital Pembrokeshire&Derwen NHS Trust [2001] EWHC 792 (Admin)

RH v South London and Maudsley NHS Foundation Trust, [2010] EWCA Civ 1273

S v Elysium Healthcare & Secretary of State for Justice [2021] UKUT 186 (AAC)

SF v Avon and Wiltshire Mental Health Partnership NHS Trust and RB (2023) UKUT 205 (AAC)

SS v Cornwall Partnership NHS Foundation Trust (Mental Health) [2023] UKUT 258 (AAC)

TTM v Hackney [2011] EWCA Civ 4

Winterwerp v Netherlands 6301/73 [1979] ECHR Article 4

Part II
Tribunal, Law, and Practice

8 The Purpose and Function of the Mental Health Tribunal

Joanne Briggs

Introduction – What is a Mental Health Tribunal?

Every Mental Health Tribunal (MHT) is a court hearing, not a meeting, and its proceedings are as consequential as those in any Crown or County Court. But the Mental Health Tribunal is a court of law possessing unique characteristics, making it very different from the mainstream judicial system and indeed from any of the other tribunals. Every MHT has a panel of three judicial decision-makers who have each been chosen for their suitability to make decisions about detention and discharge of mental health patients: a judge, a psychiatrist, and a specialist member with something relevant to bring to the role such as a background in social work, mental health nursing or occupational therapy, or special expertise from personal experience of mental illness.

One important difference between most courts and the MHT is that, if the patient is detained in hospital, the court goes to the person rather than the other way around. Most hospitals have a room dedicated to tribunal hearings, and most hearings will happen in a tribunal room. However, if needed,, the tribunal panel can decide to convene a hearing in any suitable space where the patient can go, or to which they can be bought. For example, they can hear the case in a hospital conference room; or in a community mental health centre if the patient is in a community order and not detained in hospital, or in an OT or music room attached to a PICU or higher-care ward. They could even meet in the corridor outside the door of a seclusion room, if they think this is the best way for justice to be done. They have the broadest possible discretion to adapt the tribunal process to the needs of the person who is the focus of their interest: the detained patient.

In more recent years, and increasingly frequently, hearings take place online, on a secure video conference platform provided by the Ministry of Justice called CVP which is very like the other video conferencing systems with which we have all had to become more familiar since 2020. During the coronavirus pandemic, all tribunal hearings had to take place remotely, and it remains the case since the virus controls were removed that most tribunals are held in this way. Patients currently have the right to choose whether to have a hearing in-person or online, and the majority now choose the online process.

Paper Hearings

In December 2024, Rule 35(3) of the Procedure Rules was amended to extend to detained patients the right to ask for their cases to be considered on the papers without the need for full panel hearing. It is important to acknowledge that the panel considering cases on the basis of the written evidence alone (medical, nursing and social circumstance reports), is still required to apply the same legal tests and there will be no change in the way that the panel weigh evidence

DOI: 10.4324/9781003635543-10

and assess risk. In essence the same level of anxious scrutiny would be applied even in the absence of the parties involved, (Tribunal Procedure (Amendment No. 2) Rules 2024).

How Did the MHT Come into Being?

MHTs as we now know them came into being in 1959 and were then called Mental Health Review Tribunals. Their job was to review a decision which had already been made by the patient's treating psychiatrist, to detain the patient in hospital. This review function had previously been performed in the 20th century by formal courts at various levels, in which the judge would apply a very legalistic test to decide whether the patient was "mad", within a series of legal frameworks that used terms now considered to be deeply offensive: lunatic, idiot, imbecile, feeble-minded, or insane. Evidence from doctors on this issue was not even considered to be admissible until 1930: mental health law at the time was still a hangover from the Victorian era, a time when medical care was unreliable and unpredictable, and there were many unregulated private asylums that were being run for profit.

Like all the other tribunals which were created in the second half of the 20th century, such as those concerned with employment, special educational needs, or social care or benefits, and mental health tribunal was designed to be a quicker, easier, cheaper, and less formal way to resolve a narrow legal question that would otherwise have had to go into the formal court system. All tribunals are "creatures of statute", in other words they exist because of an Act of Parliament that defines exactly how it will be constituted and what it can do. The first Mental Health Act was passed in1959, which was replaced by the Mental Health Act 1983 (updated several times by other Acts of parliament, but still the Act in force). The MHT can only do what the Mental Health Act says it can, and nothing more. A creature of statute has a fixed purpose which is described in clear words, and it cannot lawfully stray outside that description. By contrast, a High Court judge has the "inherent jurisdiction", which is the power derived from the Crown to do anything that a monarch from past times might have wanted to do.

The range of tribunal jurisdictions is now extremely wide, covering issues as diverse as war pensions and parking fines, but the MHT is there to determine a much more profound question: about the personal freedom of someone who has been forcibly contained and prevented from exercising their free will. The right not to be unlawfully locked away is a fundamental right protected by English law, and it has deep and ancient roots in our legal system. It is a right that is also recognised in many other countries by a constitution or Bill of Rights, making it an explicit and immutable entitlement for every individual citizen of those countries. In England, this legal right predates Magna Carta and was first written about in 1166. Magna Carta itself states that:

> ...no Freeman shall be taken or imprisoned...but by lawful judgment of his peers, or by the Law of the land", and further that "no legal officer shall start proceedings against anyone on his own mere say-so, without reliable witnesses having been brought for the purpose.
>
> (Magna Carta, 1166, chp.39)

This shows that, for over 800 years, the English law has tried to prevent arbitrary incarceration. And for several centuries, the only solution was to "petition the Crown", and issue what was called a writ of "*habeas corpus*", which required the person being held against their will to be brought in front of an authority who had the power to release them.

This ancient process still has echoes in mental health tribunals that take place in hospitals all over the country every day. But MHTs are of course very different from the *habeas corpus* actions that came before the advent of modern medicine and the introduction of psychiatric treatment as a medical discipline. As a society, we recognise that people who are mentally unwell can pose a risk to themselves or to others if not therapeutically contained, and that treatment can help them. Mental health care now includes a wide range of psychological and psychopharmacological strategies: in other words, therapies, and medicines. So, at the centre of the MHT's purpose and underpinning all their decision-making is mental health medicine, particularly psychiatry, and the identification of risks arising from mental disorder that might necessitate the deprivation or restriction of a patient's liberty until they are well enough to be discharged.

As the successor to the post-1959 Mental Health Review Tribunal, the MHT has continued to develop its role, in response to the changing landscape of mental health treatment and social care. In its first 75 years, the MHRT/MHT has moved between government departments, beginning in the Department of Health as a limb of the health service provided by the NHS; then it was moved to the Department of Constitutional Affairs because its function was then perceived to be closer to other kinds of public sector regulation; then it moved on to its current home, in the Primary Tier of the Heath, Education and Social Care Chamber of the Tribunal Service. This last move brought the MHT within the same organisational structure as the other courts and tribunals, in recognition of its primary function as an arbiter of justice and fairness. By contrast, what the tribunal panel does every time it sits has changed hardly at all. The tribunal's powers have adapted following various modifications brought in by statute and by case law but has remained consistent in its broad objects.

What Does the MHT Do?

The MHT reviews in each case whether a legal deprivation or restriction of the patient's liberty is necessary. Necessity is assessed according to the likely risks to the patient's own health or safety or to other persons if the legal power were to be removed. The MHT should generally be satisfied that the use of the law is the least restrictive available alternative to manage any foreseeable risks arising from the patient's condition.

How Does the MHT Make a Decision?

Like anybody who wants to come to a rational conclusion about something, the MHT will look at all the relevant facts, weigh them up, then come down on one side or the other. When doing this, the tribunal must decide on the importance of each piece of evidence and must always bear in mind that the benefit of any doubt should be weighed on the patient's side of the argument.

Before moving on to the "how", it is important to be aware of "who", because there are two distinct categories of detained patient under the Mental Health Act, and their cases are approached very differently. The majority are detained under civil powers, and are people who have simply become so mentally unwell that they need hospital treatment. These patients are detained by powers invested by law in their consultant psychiatrist, and they can be discharged from section either by their treating psychiatrist or by a tribunal. The smaller category of patients are known as "restricted patients", and are managed using different provisions of the Mental Health Act (mainly ss.37 and 41, although some restricted patients are awaiting trial in hospital or have been transferred to hospital from prison sentences under other sections). Patients who have been detained in hospital with a restriction order have always been involved in criminal proceedings in which their mental health was relevant, and they have been deemed to be likely to pose a significant risk to the public when mentally unwell. The restriction order means that the treating psychiatrist does *not* have the power to discharge the patient from the section. Only the Secretary of State for Justice, or a specially constituted tribunal, can discharge a restricted patient. Restricted patient MHTs have a judge with special experience and training, so they can guide the panel when evaluating the higher level of risk in most restricted cases and when navigating a different set of legal principles. This chapter is focussed on civil patient tribunals, which have the same overall form and participation as the narrower, restricted category.

If a civil patient is detained in hospital, either for 28 days (s.2) or for a renewable period of 6 months (s.3) the panel can decide: (i) to discharge the section immediately; (ii) to discharge the section on a future date; (iii) not to discharge the section; or (iv) to make a formal recommendation for a limited range of purposes (for a CTO to be considered, for the patient to move between hospitals, or for the patient to have s.17 leave), then come back and decide the case again if the recommendation is not followed. If the patient is subject to a Community Treatment Order (CTO), which means they can be recalled to hospital and readmitted against their will, then the tribunal has the simple power to discharge the CTO, making the patient informal in the community.

Formal recommendations ((iv) above) are made very rarely, because if the recommendation is not followed, then there ought to be some action that the tribunal could take in response, in other words, discharging the patient. But if in reality the risks to the patient or to other people would be too high to discharge, regardless of whether or not the recommendation was followed, then it is probably wrong in principle to make a recommendation in the first place.

In relation to (iii), above, "discharge on a future date", this is often referred to incorrectly, and by people who ought to know better, as a "deferred" or "delayed" discharge. Deferred discharge is a vastly different legal concept, which applies only to the smaller category of restricted patients (see above).

A discharge on a future date is not deferred because the panel must agree on a specific date and time when discharge of the section will take effect *and the section will automatically come to an end at that point.* Discharge on a future date can only be used where the panel is satisfied that there is a risk today that will be ameliorated by a significant change in circumstances, which they have been told will happen on the day that they choose: for example, if the patient would be likely to sleep on the street if she did not have any accommodation, and accommodation will become available for her on the Monday after the hearing, then the panel could exercise its discretion to discharge her on Monday at 10 am. This would be supported by a finding that being street homeless would be likely to be detrimental to her mental health and safety.

Who Can Apply to the Tribunal?

The patient can apply once in every period of detention. But in addition to patient's own applications, the Mental Health Act requires a detaining hospital to refer the patient's case to the tribunal if a certain amount of time has elapsed without them approaching the tribunal themselves. This is to make sure that all patients have the opportunity for an independent review of their situation. The Act also allows a patient's nearest relative some limited opportunities to apply. The "nearest relative" is the person nearest to the top of a list which is set out in the legislation, and they can apply to the hospital for their relative to be discharged, and then have their detention reviewed by the tribunal.

Part 1: The Beginning – What will Happen at the Tribunal Hearing?

Before the hearing takes place, the panel members review the paperwork and may form an opinion about what the issues in the case are likely to be. Sometimes the patient's case is less easy to define than the views of the professionals, as the patient's voice is communicated second-hand in quotes from clinical interviews or other situations. Occasionally, a legal representative will prepare a statement on their client's behalf or will file a position statement setting out what the main points are that they will be putting forward. In a minority of cases there is also independent expert evidence provided from the patient's side, usually from a psychiatrist instructed to challenge the treating doctor's opinion or less commonly from a psychologist or independent social worker where the patient has specific needs that may need to be met outside hospital if they were to be discharged. All of this information is evidence, so quite a lot of evidence is already in the minds of the panel members before they meet to discuss the case on the day.

Is the written evidence adequate? It is true that some reports are better than others, and some report writers are better at it, or have more time, or greater experience to bring to the task. The framework for the statutory reports (the medical, social circumstances and nursing reports that are required in every case involving a detained in-patient) is set out in a document called the **Practice Direction 2019**, which is a set of drafting requirements imposed by the most senior judge in the tribunal. The Practice Direction specifies the minimum contents of each type of statutory report, in exhaustive lists which can and probably should be followed by report writers. In practice, they rarely are, and there is usually something missing from the list in any document. A few reports can be hard to read, because they are cut and pasted from elsewhere, they have been poorly drafted, or they simply do not answer your questions. In these circumstances, MHT panel members might be within their rights to send the reports back or otherwise insist that they be done properly, complying with every letter of the Practice Direction. Occasionally, a legal representative will say that because one or more reports does not comply with the Practice Direction, the hearing should not proceed. Of course, the Practice Direction exists in the context of a larger procedural framework, the Tribunal Rules.

The Overriding Objective in Rule 2 is to **deal with cases fairly and justly**, by ensuring that the parties can participate fully in a process which is not unduly formal, overly complicated, time-consuming, or unnecessarily delayed. To give effect to the intention in Rule 2, Rule 5 gives the tribunal the power to do a wide range of things that can make the process easier, including extending or shortening time limits for things to be done, putting a case off to another day, and hearing more than one case at the same time. In particular in this instance, Rule 7 allows the tribunal to ignore a failure to comply with a Rule, or to take steps to enforce compliance. Either can be an important tool when the aim is achieving justice and fairness.

If you are a panel member, or imagine yourself in that role: do you think you should enforce compliance with the Practice Direction, if to do so will cause delay in the case? Or do you think it would it be more helpful to ask questions during the hearing instead, to fill the gaps in your understanding, and perhaps give the witness some supportive advice about following the guidance in the Practice Direction? Not everyone would necessarily agree, but I think the latter course is almost always the one that accords with the overriding objective in Rule 2: I think it fosters a good-natured atmosphere which is likely to be more reassuring for a nervous patient, and it promotes goodwill among professionals, which is beneficial for the long-term smooth running of the tribunal.

Has There Been a Pre-Hearing Examination?

Patients have the right to see the medical member of the MHT panel in private before the hearing takes place, although most will have had to apply before a procedural time-limit to exercise it. This meeting, known as a Pre-Hearing Examination (PHE), will often take place on a different day, and is frequently held on a videoconference platform such as Microsoft Teams.

The medical member will tell the other panel members about this meeting during the panel's pre-hearing preparation. That discussion will draw together the panel's preliminary views and help them to focus on what is actually in dispute, and what needs to be decided by them.

It is unusual for a patient to be unrepresented, as MHT representation is one of the few remaining areas of automatic legal aid funding, and after the Judge's introduction the patient's legal representative will probably set out in a few sentences what it is that their client wants the tribunal to do. If the patient is not represented, and the panel is content that they do not lack the necessary capacity to be so, then the panel judge will often take the lead in asking them questions, to establish what they want from the tribunal and to help them put their case. Cross examination is not necessary in a tribunal due to its inquisitorial nature, provided that there is a fair opportunity for all sides to be listened to and their point of view considered.

Where there has been a PHE, the panel judge will summarise what was said to the other panel members by the medical member at the panel's pre-hearing discussion, so the content of the PHE will then become the first piece of evidence in the hearing.

Part 2: The Middle – What will Happen at the Tribunal Hearing?

While the panel is gathering all the evidence they need from each of the witnesses according to the running-order set out by the judge in their introduction, the panel, and particularly the judge, must also keep the tribunal process running smoothly and deal with anything unexpected. The expectation at the hearing is that people do not talk over each other or out of turn, as everyone will be given a fair opportunity to say what is needed.

It is possible to predict that certain issues are likely to arise in a MHT hearing, and these have helpfully been addressed in a published set of Rules, with legal force (although less than an Act of Parliament). In this section I have summarised the rules that are used most frequently, and highlighted the general benefit the rule usually brings to the tribunal process: but I would recommend looking at the details of the Rule itself if you ever need to use and apply it. These issues can arise at any time in the process, and some are more likely than others to be raised at the beginning of the hearing, but this is an issue-based list which I hope will slot into the frame of understanding of a hearing that runs from beginning to end in the way described in the judge's introduction.

Does the Tribunal Need to Find out if the Paperwork is all in Order Before They Start?

Rule 32 governs the details of procedure in mental health cases. It is worth remembering that the MHT will not review or determine procedural irregularities unless they are (i) patently obvious; and (ii) likely to be fatal to the case because of lack of jurisdiction to continue. Most procedural irregularities can be repaired if they need to be by using Rule 5, and Rule 2 encourages pragmatism, a can-do attitude, in the interests of doing justice efficiently and expeditiously.

Who Should Have Been Told That the Hearing is Taking Place?

Rule 33 requires that notice of the case is given to a legal guardian, the Court of Protection if it is already involved with the patient's situation, the nearest relative (unless a patient with capacity objects), and any other person who the MHT thinks should be heard.

Do All Cases Have to be Decided by a Full Panel at a Hearing with Witnesses?

All tribunal applications and references will result in a hearing, provided that they are not withdrawn, and not dealt with under the fast-track procedure in Rule 35. This applies to cases referred to the tribunal concerning a community patient over the age of 18, who has said in writing that they do not wish to attend or be represented at a hearing. These cases are concluded by a single judge without a panel, based on the papers alone.

Representation, or the Lack of it

Rule 11 states that any patient, including a child, can appoint a representative; in practice nearly all representatives are legal representatives, because public funding is available to pay them. Under Rule (11)(7)(a) the tribunal can appoint a representative for someone who does not have one but would like to be represented. Under Rule 11(7)(b) the tribunal can also appoint a representative for a patient who lacks capacity, if they think it would be in their best interests. This second power is seen more frequently in action in the tribunal than the first, because it is used to protect the interests of a patient who is or has become too unwell to make rational decisions about presenting their case. If a solicitor is appointed under this provision, they must be on the Law Society's list of approved mental health lawyers, so they will be a specialist in this field of law and experienced in dealing with mentally disordered clients. A Rule 11(7)(b) appointee does not act on instructions but will often act according to the patient's expressed wishes and feelings as well as "repairing their incapacity" by acting in the client's best interests: this may include withdrawing an application on their behalf, if they think it is contrary to the patient's interests to continue (see below: Withdrawals).

What if There is Evidence That Should not be Seen by Everybody?

Rule 14 governs non-disclosure of documents or other information and is almost always used in cases where something written in a report is likely to cause a person serious harm if disclosed, and where it is also in the interests of justice to prevent its disclosure. It is quite common for this Rule to come into play to prevent disclosure to the patient of something said to the team by a close relative, but it can be engaged by covert medication regimes, or by child or adult Safeguarding investigations. The Rules and case law have shaped the process to be adopted to make a non-disclosure decision. Risk of serious harm is a high bar to get over, although the test for harm is the same as that adopted in the family courts and includes serious emotional or psychological harm.

What About Rules of Evidence, Like Hearsay?

Unlike the mainstream civil and criminal court systems, there are no rigid rules of evidence in the MHT. Rule 15 makes it clear that the form, written or oral, and the source, direct or indirect, of any evidence is up to the tribunal to decide. The MHT is inquisitorial, so the panel does not have to wait passively for each side to make an argument or establish a point in evidence. They can actively seek the material they need to make a decision and decide what weight to attach to what they see and hear when they make their decision. For completeness, Rule 34 provides the legal right to a PHE, discussed above, which is also evidence in the case. Rule 36 describes the panel's wide discretion to direct to what extent any person attending should take part in the hearing. Rule 38 empowers the tribunal panel to exclude any person if they are likely to disrupt the hearing, their presence is likely to stop someone else from being able to speak freely, or if their presence would defeat a non-disclosure direction or any other purpose of the hearing. Rule 38 also provides that all MHT hearings are held in private unless it has been directed that all or part of the hearing will be in public. There is a separate procedure for making this decision, which is part of the judicial case management undertaken by salaried mental health judges.

What if the Patient Doesn't Come to the Hearing?

If the patient does not attend, under Rule 39 the tribunal can go ahead in the patient's absence if the panel is satisfied that they know about it, they have decided not to come or are too unwell to do so, and carrying on with the hearing is in the interests of justice. This rule is most commonly used where a patient's case has been referred to the tribunal, but the patient themselves does not wish to play any part in the process.

Can the MHT Force a Witness to Come and Give Evidence?

Rule 16 gives the MHT, in theory, the power to summon witnesses to give evidence. In practice, a summons issued under this Rule would be extremely difficult to enforce, because the MHT is a creature of statute, and the Act has not given it any enforcement powers of its own. Any tribunal considering issuing a summons should consider first: is there another way to get the information we need? And if not, is there a better way to encourage or persuade the witness to provide the information they have?

What If the Patient Does Not Want the Case to Carry On?

Rule 17 allows an application to be withdrawn, either in advance or at the hearing itself. The MHT must accept the application to withdraw for it to take effect, so there is a discretion to be exercised. Recent case law has directed the MHT to ask itself the question: from what we know, are we satisfied that it is necessary to conduct a review of the patient's case? I think this means that the MHT would need to foresee a real likelihood that carrying on with the case would result in a change in the patient's legal status, in other words, discharge from section. It is very unlikely that a representative would present a withdrawal application if there was a strong or even realistic chance of discharge, so acceptance will usually follow. If the purpose of the Rules is to promote the rights and interests of the patient, (the person least able to protect their rights and interests for themselves), then it is almost always fair and just to allow that person to retain their right of application so they can use it in the future, on another, perhaps better day. There are some commentators on this Rule who cite an older case in which it was suggested that withdrawal should be refused where it "is merely a tactical ploy". For my own part, I think a "ploy" designed to keep a person detained in a hospital against their will would strain the definition of "tactical" to its limits. Such commentators have also failed to read the whole sentence in the case where this phrase appears: "…merely a tactical ploy **and is not in the interests of the patient**". It is hard to imagine a situation where wasting a patient's application, contrary to their wishes, and leaving them without a right of application until the next period of detention would be "in the interests of the patient".

Can the MHT Make an Order for Costs?

In other courts and some tribunals, it is common to talk about legal costs being paid by one side or the other, because they have lost or behaved badly in the case. Rule 10 makes it clear that in the MHT it is virtually impossible to make an order for costs. The circumstances in which you could are so unlikely to happen in an MHT that the idea can be completely discounted.

Part 3: The End and Afterwards – What will Happen at the Tribunal Hearing?

Once the evidence and submissions are over, the panel will withdraw (or if it is an in-person hearing, the witnesses will go out, leaving the panel in the hearing room), and then decide the outcome. In a minority of cases, there is insufficient evidence to make a final decision, and in these circumstances the panel has the power to adjourn, in other words to put the case off to another day and ask for more evidence to be provided by the parties in the meantime. It will usually have been evident that this evidence is missing before the hearing started, for example an important report or a live witness is not available; if that had been the case, then the better course would have been to establish whether the evidence is really absolutely necessary, and if so, to have adjourned before starting. If the case has not started, then a different panel can hear it on the next occasion, which makes relisting quicker and more efficient.

If the panel has heard evidence then the case is called "part-heard", so the same panel members should come back to finish the case at the adjourned hearing. This can put pressure on people's diaries, and finding another suitable date can be difficult if the panel does not agree on one before they leave that day.

If, as is usually the case, there is sufficient evidence to decide, then the panel will often have a discussion in which they answer the questions raised by the statutory framework for detention, by reference to particular parts of the evidence in the case: does the patient have a mental disorder? If so, is it of a nature that makes treatment in hospital necessary? And so on. If this approach is followed, it is extremely rare for there to be a fundamental disagreement about the outcome, because any difference of opinion along the way can be focussed on and ironed-out if possible. In the event that one of the panel members disagrees with the opinion of the other two in relation to the ultimate issue, detention, or discharge, then the view of the majority is the view of all three: there is no provision for one member to have a "dissenting judgment", so their opposition is put on one side. This is because, again, the MHT is a creature of statute: whereas appeal court judges are individuals sitting in a group, an MHT panel is created by law as a "three-headed" judicial decision maker with only one mind and voice with which to make and express decisions. This position may change, but it would require an authoritative statement of the law to bring it about.

When the decision has been made, it will usually be announced to the parties, unless there is a risk of the panel's delivery of a disappointing outcome resulting in extreme distress or disruption. On very rare occasions, a disappointed patient who has been given the decision in the tribunal room may become angry or aggressive. Tribunal panels should remember to do everything they can to prevent any harm being caused by the exercise of their important legal function. The room specifications for a tribunal hearing consider the need for staff to have sufficient space to manage the patient safely. This rare but real possibility underlines the need to have regard to the hospital's guidance about risks potentially arising in any hearing and considering using powers of exclusion or hearing in absence when they may be needed.

The panel's written decision contains the details of the decision they announced on the day. It must be sent to the tribunal office so it can be delivered promptly to the parties, and is always presented on a typed form, which has a logical structure to guide both the panel members and the end-users. There are time-limits for delivery (three days for S.2, and seven days for other sections), so the judge will usually draft the decision and reasons within a day or two of the hearing then email it to the other two members for their views.

If the patient was a person with a learning difficulty then an Easy Read decision can be prepared for them, with a simplified layout and language, and images to support comprehension. Easy Read decisions are written for the tribunal by an outside agency with relevant expertise in communication.

After the Hearing – Appeals and Reviews

There is a system for appealing or reviewing an MHT decision if any party to it is not satisfied with the outcome, and particularly with how the decision was reached. Being appealed is not a personal criticism of what the panel did on the day, and it is a necessary part of a fair system of open justice. If the written reasons contain a drafting error or other slip or omission which does not affect the decision reached, then this can be corrected by issuing a new decision under Rule 44. If the decision itself has been challenged, then the person asking for the whole decision to be set aside must explain why this should be done: they have to establish that there has been an "error of law" of sufficient significance that the decision cannot stand. The commonest grounds for this are that the narrative account drafted by the judge do not sufficiently explain why one side succeeded in the case and the other did not, which is called "inadequacy of reasons".

Conclusion

It has been consistently the case for many years that a very small percentage of patients are discharged by civil tribunals (although the position is slightly different for restricted patients, who can't be discharged by their treating doctor so are reliant on the tribunal or the Secretary of State to direct their discharge from hospital). An even smaller proportion of tribunal decisions is successfully overturned on appeal. I think this shows that the vast majority of in-patient treating teams have a good understanding of the balance of risk against the right not to be unnecessarily detained. And that tribunal panels act as an important check in the few cases where the balance could be struck differently, in favour of the patient's liberty.

References

Department of Health (2015). *Mental Health Act 1983: Code of Practice*. London: The Stationary Office.
Magna Carta (1166) Chapter 39.
Mental Health Act (1959). *DOH*. London: Stationery Office.
Mental Health Act (1983). *DOH*. London: Stationery Office.
Mental Health Act (1983). Sections 2, 3, 17, 37, 47. *DOH*. London: Stationery Office.
Practice Direction (2019). *First-Tier Tribunal – Health, Education, and Social Care*.
Rule 2 The Overriding Objective The Tribunal Procedure (First-tier Tribunal (Health, Education and Social Care Chamber) Rules 2008 UK Statutory Instruments No. 2699 (L. 16) London: Stationery Office.
The Tribunal Procedure (First-tier Tribunal (Health, Education and Social Care Chamber) Rules 2008 UK Statutory Instruments No. 2699 (L. 16). London: Stationery Office.
The Tribunal Procedure (Amendment No. 2) Rules 2024, UK Statutory Instruments, 2024 No. 1283 (L. 20). London: Stationery Office.

Part III
Evidence in Brief

9 Giving Evidence at the Tribunal

Kristian Garsed

Introduction

The Mental Health Tribunal is a statutory tribunal jurisdiction contained within the First-tier Tribunal, which was created by the Tribunals, Courts, and Enforcement Act 2007 and which has some characteristics, that significantly distinguish it from other jurisdictions, in particular the Criminal Courts, and most other Civil jurisdictions. As set out below, it is anticipated that the patient will be legally represented, and very rare for the Responsible Authority to have any legal representation. Next, the formal law of evidence does not apply, and instead the Tribunal has **procedural rules** which provide a very broad and generous discretion to the Tribunal in relation to the provision of evidence. Furthermore, the Tribunal is what is known as an "expert tribunal", with the decisions made by a panel appointed to the Tribunal based on specialist knowledge and expertise, which they are required to apply to the matter before them, including the evidence received. As highlighted:

> There are two particular features of tribunals and inquiries which inform the approach of the courts to the review of their functions. First, most operate on the premise that at least one of the parties is likely not to be legally represented, so that informality is at the heart of their operation, in so far as this does not conflict with the needs of justice. The formal law of evidence does not apply. Secondly, the members of the tribunal or inquiry are very often appointed either pursuant to a statutory requirement or to a general policy because they have some specialist knowledge or expertise in relation to the matters, they are likely to hear. Where they do possess this, they are expected to use it.
>
> (Expert Evidence, 2020, p.20-001)

The composition of a Mental Health Tribunal panel, as a specialist and expert Tribunal, is set out paragraph 4 of the Practice Statement "Composition of Tribunals in relation to matters that fall to be decided by the Health, Education and Social Care Chamber on or after 18 January 2010" issued by the Senior President of Tribunals on 16 December 2009. The practice statement requires that any final decision, or any decision determining any preliminary issue, at a hearing for a mental health case, must be made by the following: one judge, one member who is a registered medical practitioner, and one other member who has substantial experience of health, or social care matters. The three fields of professional experience and expertise brought together then to form this specialist and expert Tribunal are the law, medicine and medical practice, and health and social care. Professional witnesses should bear this closely in mind when preparing their written evidence or providing oral evidence to the Tribunal. Time and effort should not be wasted in an incorrect assumption that the Tribunal are not going to be able to understand or

DOI: 10.4324/9781003635543-12

apply professional evidence without precise and basic explanation of the terms, principles, or conclusions being described.

The procedural rule governing the Tribunal's powers and discretion in relation to the provision of evidence in Tribunal proceedings, is r. 15 of the Tribunal Procedure Rules 2008 (the Rules). Which sets out:

Evidence and submissions
15.—

(1) Without restriction on the general powers in rule 5(1) and (2) (case management powers), the Tribunal may give directions as to—
    (a) issues on which it requires evidence or submissions;
    (b) the nature of the evidence or submissions it requires;
    (c) whether the parties are permitted or required to provide expert evidence, and if so whether the parties must jointly appoint a single expert to provide such evidence;
    (d) any limit on the number of witnesses whose evidence a party may put forward, whether in relation to a particular issue or generally;
    (e) the manner in which any evidence or submissions are to be provided, which may include a direction for them to be given—
        (i) orally at a hearing; or
        (ii) by written submissions or witness statement; and
    (f) the time at which any evidence or submissions are to be provided.
(2) The Tribunal may—
    (a) admit evidence whether or not—
        (i) the evidence would be admissible in a civil trial in England and Wales; or
        (ii) the evidence was available to a previous decision maker; or
    (b) exclude evidence that would otherwise be admissible where—
        (i) the evidence was not provided within the time allowed by a direction or a practice direction;
        (ii) the evidence was otherwise provided in a manner that did not comply with a direction or a practice direction; or
        (iii) it would otherwise be unfair to admit the evidence.
(3) The Tribunal may consent to a witness giving, or require any witness to give, evidence on oath, and may administer an oath for that purpose.

(The Tribunal Procedure, 2008, p.84)

As can be seen from the several subsidiary provisions within Rule 15, the Tribunal has an enormously broad range of options in terms of determining; what evidence and upon what issues, evidence is required, the nature (or form) that evidence takes, whether expert evidence is necessary and how that should be organised by the parties, the quantity of evidence to be provided in particular the number of witnesses a party can be allowed to rely upon, the admissibility or inadmissibility of any potential evidence, and whether or not evidence received will be given upon oath.

In terms of that latter option, in practice the Tribunal very rarely, if ever, requires oral evidence from a professional or a lay witness, to be given on oath. It is, however, of course expected by the Tribunal that any person providing written or oral evidence to the Tribunal, whether they are a professional witness or not, will be truthful in the evidence they give. Deliberately false evidence could amount to an offence of perjury under s.1 or s.1A of the Perjury Act 1911 (depending on whether the false statement was in sworn or unsown evidence). Additionally, any dishonesty on the part of a witness could otherwise amount to contempt of court and for a professional witness who is a member of a registered and regulated health or care profession, it could also be considered as serious professional misconduct which could impair that professional's fitness to practise, and so, could require and result in a fitness to practise referral being made to the relevant professional regulatory body.

It is particularly important to note that r. 15 (2) (a) and (b) enable the Tribunal to admit, and therefore consider and apply, any evidence whether or not that evidence would be admissible in civil proceedings within the jurisdiction, and a corresponding power to exclude any evidence either due to a procedural failing, or because it would otherwise be unfair to admit that evidence. r. 15 (2) (a) and (b) are the provisions which explicitly disapply the formal law of evidence. This essentially gives the Tribunal an unlimited discretion to admit or refuse to admit any evidence, subject to the requirements of fairness and natural justice, formalised in r.2 (the overriding objective).

What is Being Decided?

The Tribunal will have to decide in accordance with r. 15 what evidence is required in order to enable the Tribunal to determine all of the issues which it must decide upon. The issues it has to resolve are first and foremost of course, the statutory criteria for detention set out in s.72 of the Mental Health Act 1983. The Tribunal may, however, have to determine other preliminary or subsidiary issues, or particular matters of fact as well, in reaching the substantive decision, applying the s.72 criteria. In *AM v Partnerships in Care Ltd* [2015] UKUT 659 (AAC)M, [2015] MHLO 106 the Upper Tribunal did not accept an argument made by the Responsible Authority which was that the Tribunal could make findings about future risk when determining whether the statutory criteria, on the basis of unproven allegations and that therefore no findings of fact were required. The Upper Tribunal instead held that although the making of decisions on the discharge criteria involves mixed questions of fact, and judgment or evaluation, the judgment or evaluation of what is likely to occur must be based on findings of fact.

In determining every issue on which it must decide then, the Tribunal has to apply the civil standard of proof, and the criminal standard of proof does not have any application in Tribunal proceedings, (R (AN) v MHRT, 2005). The issues the Tribunal has to decide are first and foremost the relevant statutory criteria under consideration in the particular case, but also (in order to inform the Tribunal's decisions on the criteria), any matter of fact asserted by the Responsible Authority or its witnesses, but which is disputed by any other party or their witnesses.

The criminal standard of proof is of course "beyond a reasonable doubt", which requires a criminal court to be "sure" on the evidence received of a defendant's guilt.

The civil standard of proof however, being "on the balance of probabilities", requires only that the Tribunal has to be satisfied in determining the issues it must decide upon, that they are probably made out, namely, they are more likely than not, on the evidence available to the Tribunal, to be met. Up until 2001 the Tribunal was only required to discharge a patient if it could be satisfied that the criteria for detention were not met, (S.72 Mental Health Act 1983). However, this ultimately had the effect of putting the burden of proof on the patient, requiring them to satisfy the Tribunal that they should be discharged. This position has now been found to be in breach of Article 5 (the right to liberty and security) of the European Convention on Human Rights, (R (H) v MHRT North and East Region [2001] EWCA Civ 415).

Instead, the current position is instead that it is for the Responsible Authority to prove that the criteria are met, in order for the Tribunal to be satisfied that the Patient should not be discharged.

The wording of the statutory criteria was amended by sections 3 and 4 of the Mental Health Act 1983 (Remedial) Order 2001, (Mental Health Act 1983 (Remedial Order 2001). The position now is that the presumption is that the patient is to be discharged from detention unless the Tribunal is satisfied that they should not be.

Evidence in the Context of the Tribunal

The *Shorter Oxford English Dictionary* provides a general definition of evidence as being: "Facts or testimony in support of a conclusion, statement or belief ... something serving as proof.", (*Oxford English Dictionary* Fifth Edition p. 875). A legal use definition is also provided as being:

> Information (in the form of personal or documented testimony or the production of material objects) tending or used to establish facts in a legal investigation ... [or] material admissible as testimony in a court of law.
>
> (Oxford English Dictionary, 2002)

Evidence, quite straightforwardly, is therefore all about proof. Evidence is no more complicated than being something which is produced in order to prove something as a matter of fact, or conversely to disprove something.
And what is proof:

> ...proof is the establishment of ... facts by proper legal means to the satisfaction of the court, and in this sense includes disproof ... Proof, apart from argument and inference drawn from facts in evidence, is effected by (a) evidence, (b) presumptions and (c) judicial notice.
>
> (Phipson, 2023, p.1-01)

Written Evidence – Senior President's Practice Direction

On 28 October 2013, Sir Jeremy Sullivan, then Senior President of Tribunals, issued the "Practice Direction First-tier Tribunal Health, Education and Social Care Chamber, Statements and Reports in Mental Health Cases", (www.judiciary.uk/wp-content/uploads/2022/09/sta tements-in-mental-health-cases-hesc-28102013.pdf), commonly referred to as "the Senior President's Practice Direction", or sometimes "the October 2013 Practice Direction". The Senior President's Practice Direction applies to all "mental health cases" as defined in Rule 1(3) the Tribunal Procedure Rules 2008 and sets out the detailed requirements for the contents of all documents which are required to be provided to the Tribunal, under r.32.

Rule. 32 sets out the requirement that particular statements and reports must be sent or delivered to the Tribunal (and, in restricted cases, to the Secretary of State) by the Responsible Authority, the Responsible Clinician, and any Social Supervisor.

The Senior President's Practice Direction is divided into five sections, covering; inpatients (both non-restricted and restricted), community patients, guardianship patients, conditionally discharged patients, and patients who are under the age of 18.

For all in-patients, the Senior President's Practice Direction stipulates that the Responsible Authority must provide (by "sending or delivering"), the following written evidence or information within 3 weeks of the application or reference being made or received by the Responsible Authority, or in s.2 cases 'as soon as practicable after receiving a copy of the application or a request from the Tribunal", (Senior President's Practice Direction, October 2013a):

- A Statement of Information about the Patient.
- A Responsible Clinician's Report, including any relevant forensic history.
- A Nursing Report, with the patient's current nursing plan attached.
- A Social Circumstances Report including details of any Care Pathway Approach.
- (CPA) and/or Section 117 aftercare plan in full or in embryo and, where appropriate, the additional information required for patients under the age of 18, and any input from a Multi-Agency Public Protection Arrangements (MAPPA) agency or meeting, (Senior President's Practice Direction, October 2013b).

Paragraph 10 of the Senior President's Practice Direction contains the important general requirements that:

- "The authors of reports should have personally met and be familiar with the patient.
- If an existing report becomes out-of-date, or if the status or the circumstances of the patient change after the reports have been written but before the tribunal hearing takes place (e.g. if a patient is discharged, or is recalled), the author of the report should then send to the tribunal an addendum addressing the up-to-date situation and, where necessary, the new applicable statutory criteria."

Paragraph 12 of the Senior President's Practice Direction includes the details of what is required for the Responsible Clinician's Report for in-patients, and paragraphs 13 and 14, the equivalent requirements for the in-patient nursing report and the in-patient social circumstances reports, respectively.

Paragraphs 18 and 19, 23 and 24, 32 and 33 contain the corresponding requirements for the Responsible Clinician's and Social Circumstances reports for community patients, Guardianship patients, and Conditionally Discharged patients, respectively. Finally, paragraph 35 sets out a series of particular additional requirements for any Social Circumstances Report, prepared for a patient who has not reached the age of 18.

Some of the principles or requirements which are to be met (which are set out in paragraphs 12, 13, 14, 23, 24, 32, and 33, in the preparation of these requisite reports are common to all three professional perspectives and for all categories of patient, in particular that:

- The report must be up-to-date, specifically prepared for the tribunal, and have numbered paragraphs and pages.
- It should be signed and dated.
- The sources of information for the events and incidents described must be made clear.
- The report should not recite the details of medical records or be an addendum to (or reproduce extensive details from) previous reports.
- In relation to the patient's current in-patient episode, the report must briefly describe the patient's current mental health presentation.

Each of the relevant paragraphs of the Practice Direction also contains what is in essence a structured index or outline of the specific and comprehensive information requirements which must be met in the proper preparation of these reports, each of which concludes with the requirement of the provision of any recommendations to the Tribunal, with reasons. It is not the intention to reproduce each of those sequences of detailed requirements here, however, what must be highlighted is that any professional witness charged with the responsibility of preparing a written report to be provided to the Tribunal, and relied upon by the Responsible Authority, must have a confident understanding of what should be, and almost as importantly, what should not be included in the report, by direct and faithful reference to the requirements of the Senior President's Practice Direction.

It really cannot be overemphasised, that this is the fundamental basis upon which witnesses written evidence, delivered to the Tribunal as a professional responsibility, must be prepared, authored, and provided. In addition to the expectations regarding the particular forms of written evidence which the Responsible Authority must provide to the Tribunal, the timescales, and the extent and quality of the information to be provided in each type of report from each particular professional, and for each category of patient, which are laid out in the Senior President's Practice Direction, there are further requirements relating to the provision of written evidence, the timeframes for that, and the consequences of non-compliance, which are contained in "The First-tier Tribunal Health, Education and Social Care Chamber (Mental Health) Enforcement Procedure, Directions and Summonses" statement, published on 24 July 2017, by M. Hinchcliffe, then Deputy Chamber President, (Practice Guidance on Enforcement Procedure).

Professional Duties and Responsibilities (Written Evidence)

Fundamentally, the provision of a written report to the Tribunal is an aspect of a designated professional's responsibilities as members of one of the registered and regulated health and care professions in the United Kingdom. Therefore, for a professional completing a written report for the Tribunal, they must as already set out, meet the standards of quality and sufficiency in terms of the information to be provided, which are described in the Senior President's Practice Direction, but in doing so each professional must also be carrying out this task, as a professional duty.

The author of the report must also have undertaken proper consideration of whether they are in fact a suitable person in terms of professional qualification, registration, and scope of practice, to provide the report at all. The fulfilment of any professional duty must be undertaken in proper observance of the standards of professional practice and behaviour, set out in the professional standards published by each of the relevant health and care professional regulators. For Responsible Clinicians, or other registered medical professionals acting on behalf of the Responsible Clinician, the standards which must be followed are set out in the current edition of 'Good Medical Practice', for registered nurses, it is 'The Code: Professional standards of practice and behaviour for nurses, midwives and nursing associates' which must be followed, and for social workers it is Social Work England's 'professional standards' which are to be adhered to. The following Chapters will explore in greater detail, the importance, and implications of providing written evidence as a registered and regulated health or care professional and will go more deeply into the particular professional considerations and expectations which must be met in performing this professional function.

Providing Quality Written Evidence

Many, but not all, Responsible Authority provider organisations make use of templates for the provision of a statutory report to the Tribunal. As long as these are up-to-date and are organised correctly in terms of the requirements of the Senior President's Practice Direction, using such a template is generally encouraged by the Tribunal as it usefully structures the report and ensures that all of the necessary considerations are addressed.

When you are using a template however, you must make sure that you have considered properly and carefully what information you are being prompted to provide at each section.

The Tribunal often sees responses to template headings which are simply not addressed to what is being asked for at that point in the report. It should go without saying, but it is vital that the correct template be adopted. The Tribunal sees frequently the use of the incorrect templates, for example a community patient social circumstances report template being completed and provided when the patient is in fact an inpatient.

Beyond simply thinking about the content of the report, witnesses should also try to be of as much practical assistance to the Tribunal members as possible. For example, they need to bear in mind that the Tribunal members are likely to prepare for a hearing by making notes, and so they are likely to be assisted by being able to copy and paste key sections from reports, or it may be that the Tribunal Judge needs to reproduce parts of the report in the written decision. In order to make that possible, reports should be submitted in an electronic format which allows for text to be copied and pasted rather than as a viewable only document, such as a read only .pdf or a scanned image file.

Even more importantly, in terms of ensuring that the report assists the Tribunal, it is important to ensure that the report is concise and efficient and enables the Tribunal to clearly understand the clinician or care professional's case and position in relation to the patient's legal status under the Mental Health Act. The Tribunal will of course need to consider the relevant context, which includes the patient's personal, forensic, and mental health histories, however context whilst necessary and important, should not be the main focus of the report. Too often the Tribunal sees reports which are almost entirely background and contextual, to the exclusion of the current picture and proper engagement with the relevant criteria. The report only needs to provide a context which is sufficient and relevant to the task of the Tribunal, so it is actually unhelpful and potentially unfair to the patient, to obscure what really matters in the report, behind pages and pages of old and irrelevant information about previous admissions which have been indiscriminately copied and pasted from the patients notes.

One of the most important components of the report is the recommendation made to the Tribunal. This should be unambiguous and based on a clear rationale which properly engages with the relevant statutory criteria. It is simply not enough to state the opinion that the criteria are met, there is a need and requirement to explain why and provide cogent rationale. It is far too common for the Tribunal to be presented with a report that merely asserts that the criteria are fulfilled, without any underlying analysis or articulation of why the Tribunal should accept that assertion. For example, if arguing that the patient is a risk to themselves and others, then it is important to give concrete examples of how the incidents relied on are linked to the patients' symptoms.

It is also important to be aware that all reports will be provided to the patient's legal representative, if they have one, and to the patient as well. Therefore, the contents of the report should not be overwhelming in terms of either extent, or the language used. Necessarily there will be clinical and legal principles and terminology included in and explored in the report. As such, it may require that careful consideration is given to the use of language. It may be helpful to have complicated terms and technical concepts need to be reworded to make them more straightforward and easily understandable.

The Tribunal understands that it is not always possible to ensure that the author of the report will attend the Tribunal hearing, to provide the oral evidence for that professional perspective, further to that report. However, it is plainly optimal for that to be the case, and it is important that when whoever accepts the responsibility of writing the report will be able to attend the Tribunal and give evidence at the hearing. More generally, it is crucial for professional groups familiarise themselves with the tribunal requirements and its process so as to plan for and enable consistency in the provision of written and oral evidence.

Providing Quality Oral Evidence

Let's start this section with the absolute basics: The Tribunal hearing is the conclusion of legal proceedings considering a patient's legal status under the Mental Health Act, and potentially (and more often than not) determining whether the patient should be deprived of their liberty or not.

As already mentioned earlier in this chapter, the Tribunal is an informal Tribunal, with a considerable discretion and flexibility in how the Tribunal proceeds and the hearing is conducted. That does not mean however, that there are no formalities or conventions, and it should be remembered by all professionals that the Patient is the focus of the Tribunal's consideration, and that the Patient must be afforded maximum dignity and respect by all participants, including the Tribunal members. Given the gravity and importance of the task of the Tribunal, professionals attending to give evidence should approach their involvement with that onus on empathy and fairness for the Patient, and the proceedings considering the Patient's legal status under the Mental Health Act, firmly in mind. This means that there are some important basic considerations, which might appear to be relatively superficial or trivial, but actually they really do matter and are important for ensuring that the Patient and the proceedings are properly respected.

These include attending on time, being dressed appropriately and professionally, not eating and drinking during the hearing (other than water of course), and making sure that if attending a virtual hearing that necessary arrangements are made to ensure privacy, in a suitable room with a suitably neutral background, where the hearing will not be disturbed. In addition, mobile phone should be off, or put in on silent, as well as any other devices which could cause a distraction, such as a laptop or an iPad are logged-off or muted.

In essence it is about paying due regard and respect to the Tribunal, being professional, be completely concentrated on the hearing, and being dedicated to the hearing for its duration. There is also the expectation that all participants ensure the privacy and confidentiality of the proceedings. If giving oral evidence to the Tribunal as a professional witness but not the author of the report, it would be good practice to be familiar with and have a good understanding of the report which has been prepared and submitted by a colleague. Even if the report was to be presented by the author, it may have been written some time ago before the time of the Tribunal hearing, so re-familiarisation is still important to as to be confident in the position taken and the information provided to the Tribunal.

This may seem obvious but again it is sadly commonplace to hear professional witnesses say that they do have a copy of the report in front of them, but they have not yet had a chance to read it. The Tribunal recognises and sympathises with extraordinary pressures which health and care providers, systems, and individual staff are currently subject to, both in the NHS and in the independent health sector, however this is so fundamental and essential in terms of proper preparation for giving oral evidence, that time simply must be found to properly read and understand the report, in order to give informed oral evidence.

If at all possible, time should be set aside, prior to the hearing, to discuss the report, and in particular the recommendation made, with the author of the report so as to ensure that rather than merely being appraised of the basic information contained in the document, there is also good understand of the approach taken in choosing the information and in formulating the recommendation and the rationale which it rests upon. Of course it is possible that having read the report a slightly, or even completely, different view may be formed, this makes it even more vital to have a discussion with the author beforehand so that any differences of professional opinion is identified early, and hopefully resolved, before any oral evidence is given to the Tribunal.

It is worth keeping in mind that the Tribunal members would have already read the report which has been provided in preparation for the Tribunal, and already have an awareness of the professional perspective, therefore, every effort should be made to avoid providing oral evidence further to that report, by simply restating the contents of the report.

The reports will however, inevitably and to various extents, be somewhat out of date by the time of the Tribunal. So there will need to be a material update, which completes the picture between the date of the report and the date of the Tribunal. The key consideration here is materiality. The update should be limited to the new information which the Tribunal needs in order to be properly informed in reaching their decision. The update absolutely does not need to cover every single clinical event or decision which has arisen in the intervening period. Witnesses are prompted or requested at the very beginning of their evidence to provide an update. If no such request is made, then it may well be that no update is considered particularly necessary. But it may be helpful to offer to provide an update in an case, even if not asked to however, and the Tribunal members can of course choose to decline the offer if they do not believe that an update is required.

Order of Evidence

The patient can give their evidence either at the beginning of at the end of the Tribunal, but the medical or nursing professional, will be asked questions first by the Medical Member of the Tribunal, or possibly the Tribunal Judge. If providing the oral social circumstances evidence then almost always the questions would first be asked by the Specialist Member of the Tribunal an then the Medical Member and maybe the Judge. All three members of the Tribunal can ask you questions however, and potentially in any order.

When giving evidence it is important to listen carefully to the questions being asked and to answer them concisely and directly. It would not be viewed negatively to ask for the question to be repeated or rephrased, and again it is perfectly acceptable to refer back to the written report, to emphasis a point or recall an incident or dates of events. When responding the panel's questions, it is important not to guess or theorise.

A particularly important consideration for medical professionals, is that they are likely to be asked by the Tribunal Judge to confirm, prior to giving their oral evidence, which of the statutory criteria they are relying upon. When responding, careful and discerningly consideration should be given about which criteria are relied upon and the reasons. It is not enough to just assert that reliance is placed on all the possible criteria, the panel would expect evidence on the criteria. So, it be necessary to concede that some criteria are not relevant or will not be met. Also, the Tribunal can only make binary findings, namely that a particular criterion is, or is not met, to the Tribunal's satisfaction. The Tribunal cannot make partial or ambiguous findings, so witnesses should not seek to rely only partially or ambiguously on any particular criterion. If there is doubt or lack of confidence that a criterion is fulfilled, then it is very unlikely that the Tribunal will be able to reach a finding that it is.

Having given confirmation of the professional position in relation to the relevant criteria, there is opportunity to depart from that position during the oral evidence, if appropriate, but that should be rare and only for good reason.

Consideration of the Patient

Ideally, and good practice, the Patient should have been met and spoken to about the Tribunal hearing beforehand. The Patient should be aware of those giving evidence, as a professional witness, at the hearing. It Patient will find it difficult, understandably, to hear evidence being given about them by professionals not previously involved in their care or treatment, and who they do not know, and with whom they have no established relationship.

It would be helpful to the Tribunal and to the medical professional giving evidence to have undertaken a recent review of the Patient and ideally have completed an up-to-date mental state examination. Similarly, the nursing professional should have had some recent involvement in the care of the Patient, and, as minimum, have reviewed their nursing notes, and other records of their care and treatment.

Also, the professional giving the oral social circumstances evidence should ensure that they have met or spoken with the Patient in preparation for the hearing, and if possible have obtained an impression of their views, wishes and intentions. Just as importantly, they should also have sought, or at least attempted to ascertain, the views of the Nearest Relative if there is one.

It is worth keeping in mind that when being questioned at the Tribunal hearing, it is an exchange with the questioner and not to get drawn into a conversation or debate with the Patient, who may very well interrupt and seek to respond with their own views or challenge the responses. However, the Patient is the subject of the hearing, and it will understandably and perhaps unavoidably be a difficult experience for them to hear evidence, especially if they disagree with it.

Usurpingly perhaps, it is not in every case that there is much or anything which is in dispute. Sometimes, most commonly when the hearing is to consider a mandatory statutory reference, the Patient and their legal representative on their behalf are entirely in agreement with the position taken by the Responsible Authority and the professional witnesses or are otherwise neutral in relation to the relevant criteria. However, professional witness must still be prepared to be challenged sometimes at length, repeatedly and in microscopic levels of detail, on the evidence they have provided, and the position taken.

The Tribunal hearing is not as adversarial as compared to many other jurisdictions, however there is an element of this, and witnesses will to all intents and purposes sometimes be cross examined by a legal professional instructed by the Patient to represent their position or perhaps appointed by the Tribunal to represent the Patient's legal best interests, if they lack capacity to appoint and instruct their own representation.

When being questioned by the Patient's legal representative, the professionals being cross-examined should remain calm, objective, and focussed on the questions being asked. The stance throughout should be to remain composed, not to become agitated or irritated, and not to respond to questions by asking questions in reply. Just as when being questioned by the members of the Tribunal, the answer should be concise and direct, and with reference to the information that is available. Propositions asserted by the Patient's representative should not be accept, unless it is genuinely agreed, and questions which require hypothesise or speculations should be avoided.

Finally, in terms of consideration of the Patient, it is important to acknowledge the fact that the first and most obvious consequence of evidence not being accepted by the Tribunal, is that is very likely that the Tribunal will discharge the Patient from the section which is being considered at the hearing. Therefore professionals giving evidence must anticipate this as a possibility and ensure that if that is the decision of the Tribunal, arrangements are in place to accommodate and facilitate that decision.

Conclusion

It is noteworthy that although the Tribunal strives to create an informal atmosphere in order to keep the patient at ease and not overwhelm them with formalities, it is still a court, and all professional participants are expected to act accordingly. As such in giving written or oral evidence, the Tribunal expects all the relevant professional standards of performance and behaviour that could reasonably be expected of a registered and regulated health or care professional in all the circumstances of the case. The Tribunal could, if it so thinks fit, to make a fitness to practise referral to the relevant professional regulatory body if such course of action is deemed to be warranted. Additionally, other concerns may be identified during the provision of evidence, for example safeguarding concerns, or concerns about the provision of care or treatment, which could merit onward referral to other organisations, such as the local authority, the CQC, or the ICB. Any such concerns would need to be raised and discussed with a Duty Judge or the District Tribunal Judge for the area, to determine what further action, if any, may be appropriate or required. Of course, these situations are extremely rare, however, it does highlight the possibilities that exists and the importance for those giving evidence to be aware of their role, duties and responsibilities when appearing and giving evidence before the Tribunal.

References

AM v Partnership in Care Ltd [2015] UKUT 659 (AAC)M, [2015] MHLO 106.

Chamber Tribunal Rules. No 2699, www.gov.uk/government/publications/health-education-and-social-care-chamber-tribunal-rules (Accessed: 15 November 2024).

Expert Evidence: Law and Practice 5th Ed. 2020 – Section A. – Statutory Tribunals and Inquiries 20-001. Sweet and Maxwell Ltd, UK. www.judiciary.uk/wp-content/uploads/2022/09/statements-in-mental-health-cases-hesc-28102013.pdf.

Mental Health Act 1983 (Remedial) Order 2001.

Oxford English Dictionary 2002 (5th Ed). Oxford University Press.

Phipson on Evidence 2023 (20th Ed). Thompson, Sweet and Maxwell, UK.

Practice Guidance on Enforcement Procedure –www.mentalhealthlaw.co.uk/media/Practice_Guidance_on_Enforcement_Procedure,_Directions_and_Summonses_(24-7-17).pdf

The Tribunal Procedure (First-tier Tribunal). (2008) *Health Education and Social Care*

R (H) v MHRT North and East Region [2001] EWCA Civ 415.

R (AN) v MHRT [2005] EWCA Civ 1605).

S. 72 Mental Health Act 1983.

Senior President's Practice Direction October 2013a Paragraphs 8 and 9.

Senior President's Practice Direction October 2013b Paragraphs 7 and 8.

The Shorter Oxford English Dictionary Fifth Edition.

The Tribunal Procedure (First-tier Tribunal) (Health, Education and Social Care Chamber) Rules 2008 r. 15. 2008 No. 2699.

10 The Nursing Evidence

Helen Rees and Jennifer Oates

Introduction

The purpose of Mental Health Tribunal hearings is to provide evidence to the Mental Health Tribunal that the patient meets the legal criteria for detention. Nurses are expected to understand the various legal criteria they regularly work with. This includes: the Mental Health Act, (1983), the Mental Capacity Act, (2005), the Equality Act, (2010), and the Human Right Act, (1998). Staying up to date with relevant laws is a nursing duty outlined by the Nursing and Midwifery Council (2018):

> *17.3 have knowledge of and keep to the relevant laws and policies about protecting and caring for vulnerable people.*
>
> (Nursing and Midwifery Council 2018, p.18)

This chapter should, therefore, be read with these legislative frameworks in mind and in conjunction with Chapter 8, which outlines the legislative criteria for detention under the Mental Health Act, (1983). The registered mental health nursing role is unique, and as such, the evidence they provide is an important part of the safeguarding function of the hearing. In most inpatient environments nurses have the most sustained direct patient contact, given nursing care is 24/7, (Felton, Repper and Avis, 2018). This means that nurses have comprehensive knowledge of the patient's mental state and current degree of mental disorder. Nurses' objective recording of information about mental state and the ability to report this according to regulatory requirements is a core competency of the registered nursing roles, (Health Education England, 2020). In particular, nurses can provide significant insights about specific examples of symptoms that are documented in the medical report, the daily functioning of the patient, their medication regime and compliance, section 17 leave arrangement, incidents, insight, relationships with others, and their response to treatment. Shared decision making, co-production, and collaboration are essential foundations of person-centred, recovery-orientated nursing care. This means that the nursing report can make an important contribution to understanding if detention under the Mental Health Act, (1983) is necessary or if a less restrictive approach is possible.

Preparing the Patient for a Mental Health Tribunal Hearing

The nursing role in the hearing starts before the date directed to submit the report. Indeed, registered nurses can play a key role in making hearings accessible to patients. It is important that nurses know when patient's may be eligible to apply for a Mental Health Act Tribunal hearing or when they may be referred for one (more detail about this can be found in Chapter 8).

DOI: 10.4324/9781003635543-13

Often, hearings are discussed with patients as part of the nurse informing the patient of their rights under Section 132, (Mental Health Act Code of Practice, 2015). Nurses should be able to advise patients about what powers the Tribunal has, what evidence the Tribunal will be requesting, and that they (the patient) have a right to see any written evidence in advance (this is generally supported by their legal representative). This information can be found in the Mental Health Act Code of Practice, (2015). Patients should also be informed about their right to free legal representation; indeed nursing staff should facilitate patients access to their legal representative meetings.

The MHA Code of Practice, (Department of Health, 2015), places a duty on to clinical teams to consider the patient's welfare during the hearing. Working together to consider what support a patient may need is a way of fulfilling this duty. Nurses can increase the accessibility of the hearing by working with patients to prepare them for what will happen when evidence is given. This could include visiting the meeting space where the hearing will take place, talking about who will be present and where they will sit when oral evidence is given.

Patients must be aware that their hearing is occurring and should be given support to attend, (Department of Health, 2015). In the case of non-attendance by the patient, carrying out the outlined steps in this paragraph may support you to provide evidence that the patient is aware of the hearing and making an informed choice not to attend. When the Responsible Authority cannot provide such evidence this can increase the risk of unnecessary adjournments. It is also important that you make the tribunal aware if the patient does want to attend the hearing, but the date and time is preventing them from doing so, (for example, if they are unwell on the day).

Writing the Report

The template for writing the inpatient nursing report is published by HM Courts and Tribunal Service (2018), although some responsible authorities have their own templates for the nursing evidence. The report should reflect the views of the inpatient nursing team and wider multi-disciplinary team, however, where practicable, reports should be written in consultation with the patient. This can be done at opportunities such as planned 1:1 sessions, as part of care planning, or during a discharge planning meeting. The nursing team and patient may disagree on the content. If this is the case, then it is important to acknowledge what the disagreement is, provide evidence to support the view of the nursing team, and allow the patient to provide evidence supporting their view. Practicing in this way reduces the risk of damage to any therapeutic relationship, (Rees, 2023).

Presenting the Report

Best practice is that the nurse attending the hearing is the same nurse who wrote the report. People in charge of rostering should consider facilitating report authors to present oral evidence where possible. Given that nursing teams work shifts over a 24/7 period, it is not always possible for the same nurse to undertake both activities. Both the report writer and the presenter should know the patient well and be able to speak to the collective view of the nursing team. Where report writer and presenter differ, it is helpful if the report author gives a handover to the nurse who will give oral evidence. If the nursing recommendations are different to the others, then it is best practice to have this discussion with the other representatives (the authors of the medical and social circumstances reports) prior to the tribunal. This ensures consistency in care. It is not unusual for nursing teams to have a different view from the medical team regarding whether the criteria for detention are met, but it is concerning for the panel and potentially confusing for the patient, if this difference of opinion only becomes apparent to each party during the course of the hearing.

Inside the Hearing Room

Whether in person or remote, most likely the nurse will be sat next to the patient during the hearing. This means that you can be a source of calm and reassurance to them, you will know, from your ongoing contact with them as an inpatient, what may be triggers or warning signs of them becoming distressed. You will likely know the degree of risk to themselves or others they may present with when distressed. You may need to use your therapeutic engagement skills to help the patient remain calm and focused when listening to the evidence. In some instances you may want to ask for breaks in proceedings so the patient can calm down and refocus. It is worth noting that the panel and the other people present will be experienced with dealing with mentally distressed patient and will likely pick up on any cues that a patient needs time out. You can ask for breaks and you should be supported if you say there needs to be a break, based on your nursing expertise and knowledge of the patient.

Hearing a tribunal outcome can be distressing for the patient. Usually, after deliberations, the tribunal judge gives the outcome of the hearing but does not give detailed reasons for the decision. Those reasons will be provided in writing promptly after the hearing. If the decision is not in accord with the patient's desired outcome then this may make the patient distressed, upset or angry. It is good to have a plan in place with other nursing colleagues for how to support the patient after the tribunal. If your patient is at risk of violence and aggression then you should make a plan for how to manage that risk in the hearing room and afterwards. This could include the use of de-escalation techniques with the patient, but also considering how the physical environment of the hearing room can be made as safe as possible, for example how chairs and equipment are positioned in relation to each other and to the people in the room.

In the following we take each section of *Form T134*. We cover important considerations and principals for completing each section with regards to submitting written evidence and potential related questions from the tribunal.

Patient Details

It is important that basic information such as preferred name, date of birth, date of admission etc. are correct. Not only is this important to ensure that the tribunal members have the correct information, but the quality of the writing increases confidence in the evidence given, and demonstrates respect for a process which is of extreme importance to the patient.

Are There Any Factors That May Affect the Patient's Understanding or Ability to Cope with Hearing?

Illness and disability can impact all areas of functioning, and this may include mental state, concentration, retention, and ability to sit still for long periods of time. If the Mental Health Act Tribunal are aware of this, they are able to make reasonable accommodations to ensure the patient can fully participate. It is helpful to include in the report, for example, anything relevant about the patient's preferred name or pronouns, times of protected meals, medication times, the need for regular breaks, support arranged from an advocate, or the need for the patient to get up and walk around.

Are There Any Adjustments That the Tribunal May Consider in Order to Deal with the Case Fairly and Justly

It is important that the Mental Health Tribunal Service is given as much notice as possible about reasonable adjustments that would enable a patient to participate fully in their hearing. Adjustments may include things such as preference for a video or a face-to-face hearing, having an afternoon hearing due to morning drowsiness from medication, requiring a full day hearing to allow for the facilitation of regular breaks, and the use of interpreters. People experiencing mental and physical disorders are protected by the Equality Act, (2010). This means that clinicians have a legal responsibility to consider reasonable adjustments that allow a patient to engage with the tribunal process. Whilst many reasonable adjustments will need to be discussed with the patients' legal representative with as much notice as possible it is also important that the Tribunal panel are made aware through the report.

What Is the Nature of Nursing Care and Medication Currently Being Made Available to the Patient?

The nursing team have an oversight of the treatment that is been offered to the patient and a summary of this should be available through documented care plans. This is an important part of providing evidence that appropriate treatment is available, a key part of the legal criteria for detention.

Common areas of nursing care planning and delivery include physical health monitoring; leave monitoring; psychoeducation; activity planning; health promotion; mood monitoring; talking therapies; providing 1-1 sessions; relapse prevention; and supporting patients to write advanced statements around future care preferences, (NHS England, 2023). Providing evidence about a patient's engagement with these areas of treatment as well as their progress (or reasons for not engaging in any of these areas of care offered) will support the tribunal in understanding the current degree of illness.

Registered nurses also have responsibility for medication administration and as such can provide useful information about medication concordance and the level of care required to ensure the patient is taking prescribed medication.

Evidence around medication concordance may include things such as:

* Does the patient come to have medication at the prescribed time, or do they require prompting?
* Is there a plan or opportunity to move towards self-medication; if self-medication is already happening what is the team's assessment of how this has gone?
* How frequently are any as required medications used?

The evidence around treatment may also include feedback from other professionals who have not had the opportunity to contribute to the hearing evidence such as psychologists, occupational therapists, activity workers etc. This may be particularly important for patients who are likely to stay in hospital for long periods of time due to the risks they present when unwell. Including any assessments from the multi-disciplinary team (either completed or planned with a rough proposed timeline) can support an overall picture of the patient's progress with treatment. This report section is particularly important for Sections of the Mental Health Act, (2008), that require appropriate medical treatment to be available to meet the legislative requirement for legal detention.

To What Level of Observation Is the Patient Currently Subject?

Psychiatric observations are part of nursing care, treatment for mental disorders and support with maintaining safety and managing risk. They can range from: several members of staff needing to always be within arm reach of the patient in a low stimulus environment (such as seclusion), to needing to see the patient once within an hour. Therefore, understanding changes to the observation level and the rationale behind the clinical decision making can provide insights into the individual's progress in terms of safety and risk. Remember that naming conventions of psychiatric observations are not universal and clinical jargon should be avoided, for example, saying "within eyesight" is better understood than "level 1".

Does the Patient Have Contact with Relatives, Friends or Other Patients?

Due to the nurse's proximity to patients, they are often best placed to provide feedback on the contact the patient is having with relatives, friends, and other patients. It is important to acknowledge that patients may not always give permission to share information with their relatives and friends. If the patient does not give permission for information about them to be shared, this does not prevent the care team from seeking information about the nature of contact they are having with the patient, where appropriate, (Royal College of Psychiatrists, 2017).

Family-centred care can be important part of recovery, (Foster and Isobel, 2018). Whilst next-of-kin and other supporters do not currently have the same rights under the Mental Health Act, (2008) as the Nearest Relative, anyone in regular contact with the patient may provide valuable insights into their current mental state and premorbid personality. Positive contact with support networks can also be a significant protective factor. In addition, evidence of facilitating contact with a patient's support network can demonstrate steps taken to minimise restrictions.

Reporting on contact with support networks can also help the Tribunal consider evidence regarding any risk factors in relationships. This is important as some people who are acutely unwell experience increased vulnerability to abuse including sexual, financial, and physical exploitation (Dean et al., 2018). It is also important to find out about any caring responsibilities a patient may have. This allows any safeguarding concerns to be factored into the decision whether care could be delivered in a less restrictive environment. Information may include frequency and any changes in mental state pre, during or post-contact.

Reporting on any contact during visits or leave can also provide insights into how a patient may cope outside the relational security provided by the inpatient environment.

A mental disorder may reduce an individual's ability to engage in social interaction. This may be due to withdrawal, low self-esteem, or a difficulty in interpreting social interactions of others, (Anderson, Laxham and Priebe, 2015). Sharing relevant information about the patient's interactions with peers is a key part of the risk assessment, and can provide valuable insights into any potential vulnerability or risks to others. It is important to understand if a patient can tolerate time in other people's company or spends long periods of time isolated. Difficulties with social interaction (for instance unprompted aggression, poor anger management, and sexual disinhibition) may increase risks both for the individual and for members of the public, (Hart, 2023).

What Community Support Does the Patient Have?

Updates from the patient's network can also potentially provide insights into what support would be available to the individual in the community. This is sometimes an area of difference of opinion between patient and their support network, for example a patient may be of the view that "my family are happy for me to be cared for at home," whereas their family members may say that they do not feel comfortable or safe caring for them in their home. In such circumstances, the Nearest Relative, or other members of the support network may wish to give their view of confidence to the care team and the panel. What this means is that report writers can ask that some parts of their reports are not disclosed to the patient. There is further information about when it is appropriate to be asked for information to be withheld in the Mental Health Act Code of Practice, (2015). Understanding what community mental health services are in place or could be in place for the patient at discharge is also useful. This should include any voluntary or non-government organisations that the patient finds supportive.

What Are the Strengths or Positive Factors Relating to the Patient?

This is an opportunity to consider protective factors that may reduce the risk to the patent and strengthen areas of resilience (Ungar and Theron, 2020). This is also an opportunity to prevent the hearing problem being focused and for professionals giving evidence to demonstrate positive regard and respect towards the patient. You could comment on how the patient has coped well with challenging dynamics on your ward, or when they have shown enthusiasm for ward-based activities. You could describe their interests and motivations.

Give a Summary of the Patient's Current Progress, Engagement with Nursing Staff, Behaviour, Cooperation, Activities, Self-Care and Insight.

This section of the report is an opportunity to consider whether the patient has the skills required to maintain a good quality of life and live as independently as possible. Many people experience a reduction in their ability to manage activities of daily living when they are unwell, and it is useful to include any information the team have from prior to admission about these activities that may indicate a change in mental state.

Current progress should be supported by a summary of the individual's mental state and any marked changes to this during the admission period. This should be in a similar format to a mental state examination which is a universally recognised way of assessing someone's current level of mental distress, (Soltan, 2017).

When reporting on the patient's mental state it is essential to consider alternative explanations and provide evidence with regards to the views of the nursing staff. For instance, are signs of irritation most likely related to a mental disorder or due to being in a restrictive environment where the individual may find it difficult to have their needs met? It is also important to consider whether a stable mental state is unduly impacted upon by the relational security provided by the ward, and therefore may require further testing within the boundaries of restriction under the Mental Health Act, (1983), to minimise risk to the individual and members of the public.

Current progress should also include an update on how the patient is progressing with the care plans outlined under the nursing care section of the report. Areas of daily living that may be considered when reporting on progress, activities, and self-care include:

- Personal care (including hygiene and grooming)
- Meeting hydration and nutritional needs
- Engaging in meaningful activity
- Sleep
- Social interactions
- Budgeting.

Personal Care

Some people find that maintaining personal care becomes harder when they are mentally unwell. This may be due to symptoms such as: low motivation, paranoia, and reduced cognitive functioning (Best et al., 2020). Understanding how well someone can maintain elements of personal care can help the tribunal understand the risks to the individual's health and safety as well as give a picture of their current cognitive functioning.

- How frequently is the person washing themselves and are they able to wash themselves effectively?
- Do they require any prompt with carrying out personal hygiene and wearing clean clothes?
- Is the individual able to keep their room area clean and tidy, how much support do they require with this?
- Do they store things in such a way that it could cause a health and safety hazard – for instance large amounts of items that make it harder to exit the room in an emergency.

Remember personal hygiene needs will differ for each individual and are likely to involve important elements of the individual's personal culture. Therefore, it is important to spend time understanding if the person has everything they need to carry out personal hygiene as they wish before claiming that someone is unable to do this independently.

Carrying out home visits with the patient can provide helpful insights into how someone may function outside of an inpatient environment. This is important as an inpatient environment does not always allow individuals to practice independence with regards to personal care and therefore it can be hard to provide a picture of how someone may function (or have been functioning) prior to admission. If someone has lived with their family or in supported accommodation it is useful to get information about how they were managing to maintain their environment and the nursing team should be proactive in gaining this information.

Meeting Hydration and Nutritional Needs

Many people experiencing an acute period of mental distress have difficulties meeting their hydration and nutritional needs which are important with regards to the health and safety of the individual (Teasdale et al., 2017). The evidence in this section may take on particular importance for someone whose disorder means they are likely to act in an extreme way around food and fluid e.g. psychogenic polydipsia and anorexia nervosa.

It is important to know if someone can eat and drink within an inpatient environment but also important to consider that there are limited opportunities to demonstrate independence with regards to: budgeting, shopping for ingredients, meal preparation, safe use of kitchen equipment, and safe food preparation. It may not be safe to assess some of these in certain environments. This is why it is important when preparing for discharge to give a person the opportunity to practice these skills either as part of nursing care or working closely with other professions such as occupational therapists.

Engaging in Meaningful Activity

Engaging in meaningful activity may also be a protective factor with regards to acute mental distress. Planning and initiating an activity involve complex cognitive and communication skills and therefore if people are able to manage their time it can demonstrate progress with regards to mental state. Examples of appropriate evidence may include:

- Is the individual able to plan activities they enjoy?
- Do they have access to leave and if so are they able to use it appropriately?
- What do they do during leave, and do they return on time?
- Considering activities may also provide insights into skills such as road safety and social communication around meeting needs (e.g. make purchases in a shop).

Whilst social interaction with friends and family may be considered in other sections of the nursing report, considering activity is also an opportunity to explore the ability of the patients to build appropriate relationships with healthcare staff. Not only does this continue to provide potential insights into functioning it also helps the tribunal consider the likelihood that the patient will engage with healthcare staff upon discharge.

Sleep

Sleeping disturbances are present in a high proportion of mental disorders (Freeman et al., 2020). It is not clear if sleep disturbances are a causal or symptomatic factor of mental disorders but for some people sleep changes are an early warning sign. Therefore, understanding any changes in a person's sleeping pattern can provide useful information with regards to their mental state. The nursing team generally have a good idea of how someone is sleeping, and important information may include noting if the patient is sleeping too little or too much? The amount of sleep required will vary for each individual, however it is agreed that most people require around 7-9 a day for adults, (Hirshkowitz et al., 2015).

Budgeting

Does the patient have access to finances and are they able to spend money in a way that ensures their needs are met, for example, are they able to prioritise paying for their accommodation (mortgage or rent), utilities and food. Some mental disorders have disinhibition as a symptom which can result in excessive spending of money and cognitive difficulties can result in poor budgeting (Bond, Braveman and Clarke, 2018). Likewise, poor finances can be a sign of financial abuse and debt can be a source of distress. All of these areas present an opportunity to report on behaviour and cooperation with planned treatment both as inpatient and, while on leave.

Insight

Insight considers if the person recognises the symptoms of their illness (David, 1990). This includes understanding of why other people may have concerns about their mental state, the risks this exposes them to or the risks this exposes others to. This may include the patient's understanding of why they are detained and what they attribute any risk to.

Details of any occasion on which the patient has been absent without leave whilst liable to be detained, or occasions when the patient has failed to return when required after having been granted leave. This information is useful as it gives the tribunal an understanding of if the patient may continue to engage with mental health care on an informal basis, and therefore, could be managed in a less restrictive way. If a patient is complying with leave restrictions (or not) can contribute to understanding if a patient will continue to comply with treatment if they were discharged from the Section they are detained under.

What Is the Patient's Understanding of, Compliance with, and Likely Future Willingness to Accept Any Prescribed Medication or Treatment for Mental Disorder That Is or Might Be Made Available?

Including any expressed views and preference on medication may support the tribunal in their assessment of how likely treatment continuation is if detention is discontinued. It is also important to report on any understanding the patient has regarding what medication they take, why they take it, and what (if any) they feel the benefits are of taking it. It is important to understand that many patients report iatrogenic harm from psychiatric medication, and therefore, non-compliance cannot be considered as a sign of reduced insight in isolation, (Pearson and Pringle, 2014). Feedback on any contact with community services may help understand if the patient will engage in assessment, monitoring, and treatment if discharged from detention. Any work done on relapse prevention or early warning signs may provide evidence that a patient has an understanding of their illness and when they should seek support.

Give Details of Any Incidents Where the Patient Has Harmed Themselves or Others or Threatened to Harm Others

Assessment of risk is a key part of determining whether someone can be managed in a less restrictive environment. Risk is not static, and it should be made clear in evidence whether what is been referred to is historic or current; it is essential that risk assessments are regularly reviewed and updated (Warrander, 2024). People with dependency on substances and alcohol are at a higher risk of serious mental illness, (Public Health England, 2017). Substance and alcohol use may increase the chances of impulsive behaviour and should be considered as something that may impact risk (Callaghan and Sutcliffe, 2024). It is important the Tribunal are made aware of any drug or alcohol use and the willingness of the patient to engage in any harm minimisation work around this.

Harm to self may include incidents such as:

- Ligaturing
- Head banging
- Suicidal ideation
- Exposure to high-risk environments (either intentionally or unintentionally)
- Restriction of food or fluid
- Cutting, burning or self-poisoning
- Insertion of harmful objects
- Non-compliance with physical health medication.

Harm to others may include incidents such as:

- Abusive language (including targeted abuse aimed at an individual's characteristic, such as their gender, race, sexuality etc.)
- Aggression
- Stalking
- Violence

- Use of weapons to intimidate
- Irresponsible driving.

Give Details of Any Incidents Where the Patient Has Damaged Property, or Threatened to Damage Property

Damage to property can put others at risk as well as give an indication of the current mental state. Damage to property may include:

- Arson
- Flooding
- Kicking or hitting walls, doors or furniture items.

Understanding severity, any patterns, triggers, factors associated with thinking at the time of the incident, (e.g., cognitive rigidity), intent, level of impulsivity, and planning with all areas of risk will support the overall assessment, (Hart, 2023). It is also helpful to understand if the individual acknowledges the risks associated with their actions and whether they minimise these or take responsibility for their actions.

Have There Been Any Occasions Where the Patient Has Been Secluded or Restrained?

Incidents of seclusion and restraint can provide information about the current degree of illness. They are also restrictive, and have potential to worsen mental state and cause trauma, (Wood, McLaughlin and Owen, 2017). Including information about the frequency, how often use is reviewed and which professions are involved in the review can support the tribunal to consider if a less restrictive care option is possible.

In Section 2 Cases Is Detention Justified or Necessary in the Interests of the Patient's Health or Safety, or for the Protection of Others?

This section should present a brief summary of the salient evidence you have included and its relation to the legislative criteria.

In All Other Cases Is the Provision of Medical Treatment in Hospital Justified or Necessary in the Interests of the Patient's Health or Safety, or for the Protection of Others?

As above, this section should present a brief summary of the salient evidence you have included and its relation to the legislative criteria.

If the Patient Was Discharged from Hospital, Would They Likely Act in a Manner Dangerous to Themselves or Others?

This should be a summary of the current risk and resilience factors outlined in previous parts of the report. Any recommendation should be justified with a summary of supporting evidence.

Please Explain How Risks Could Be Managed Effectively in the Community, Including the Use of Any Lawful Conditions or Recall Powers

It is essential that discharge planning starts from admission and any update on current progress should consider steps required to facilitate discharge. Mwebe (2023), highlights that limited discharge planning can be a factor in preventing the reduction of restrictions. Reporting on how the team is supporting the patient to move towards discharge reduces the risk that a patient is detained unnecessarily due to poor provision of less restrictive options. The focus of this section should consider what would need to happen to make community management possible. Consideration should be given to any conditions that the nursing team feel would be required to facilitate this and why the power of recall is necessary if a Community Treatment Order is recommended as the least restrictive option.

Do You Have Any Recommendations for the Tribunal?

Recommendations must relate to the legal criteria and be based on the evidence already provided in the report.

Conclusion

In this chapter we have made the case that nursing evidence can provide significant insights to Mental Health Tribunals. We have outlined key areas for consideration in the provision of inpatient nursing evidence in mental health hearings. Finally, we encourage nurses to reflect on the difference they can make to ensure that patients feel supported throughout the Mental Health Tribunal process, and that evidence presented is founded on the legal criteria within the Mental Health Act (1983).

Bibliography

Akther, S. F., Molyneaux, E., Stuart, R. et al. (2019). Patients' experiences of assessment and detention under mental health legislation: systematic review and qualitative meta-synthesis. *BJ Psych Open.* 5: p. 3. doi: 10.1192/bjo.2019.19

Anderson, K., Laxham, N., and Priebe, S. (2015). Can mental health interventions change social networks? A systematic review. *BMC Psychiatry.* 15: p. 297.

Anthony, W. (1993). Recovery from mental illness. The guiding vision of the mental health service systems in the 1990s. *Psychosocial Rehabilitation Journal.* 16: p. 1123.

Best, M. W., Law, H., Pyle, M., and Morrison, A. P. (2020). Relationships between psychiatric symptoms, functioning and personal recovery in psychosis. *Schizophrenia Research.* 223: pp. 112–118.

Bond, N., Braverman, R., and Clarke, T. (2018). *Recovery Space. Minimising the Financial Harm Caused by Mental Health Crisis.* www.moneyandmentalhealth.org/wp-content/uploads/2018/02/Money-and-Mental-Health-Recovery-Space-Report.pdf [Accessed 23rd September 2024].

Callaghan, P., and Sutcliffe, A. (2024). Working with people with substance misuse problems. In: Callaghan, P., Dickinson, T., and Felton, A. (eds.) *Mental Health Nursing Skills 2e.* Oxford: Oxford University Press.

David, A. S. (1990). Insight and psychosis. *British Journal of Psychiatry.* 156: pp. 798–808.

Dean, K., Laursen, T. M., Carsten, B. et al. (2018). Risk of being subjected to crime, including violent crime, after onset of mental illness. A Danish national registry study using police data. *JAMA.* 75(7): pp. 689–696.

Department of Health. (2015). *Mental Health Act 1983: Code of Practice.* London: The Stationary Office

Felton, A., Repper, J., and Avis, M. (2018). Therapeutic relationships, risk, and mental health practice. *International Journal of Mental Health Nursing.* doi: 10.1111/inm.12430

Foster, K., and Isobel, S. (2018). Towards relational recovery: nurses' practices with consumers and families with dependent children in mental health inpatient units. *International Journal of Mental Health Nursing.* 27: pp. 727–736.

Freeman, D., Sheaves, B., Waite, F., Harvey, A., and Harrison, P. J. (2020). Sleep disturbance and psychiatric disorders. *The Lancet Psychiatry.* 7(7): pp. 628–637.

Hart, C. (2023). *A Pocket Guide to Risk Assessment and Management in Mental Health* (2nd ed.). London: Routledge.

Health Education England. (2020). *Mental Health Nursing Competence and Career Framework.* www. hee.nhs.uk/sites/default/files/documents/HEE%20Mental%20Health%20Nursing%20Career%20 and%20Competence%20Framework.pdf

Hirshkowitz, M., Whiton, K., Albert, S. M. et al. (2015). National Sleep Foundation's updated sleep duration recommendations: final report. *Sleep Health.* 1(4): pp. 233–243. doi: 10.1016/j. sleh.2015.10.004

HM Courts and Tribunals Service. (2018). *Form T134: In-Patients: Nursing Report.* www.gov.uk/gov ernment/publications/form-t134-in-patient-nursing-report. [Accessed 23rs September 2024]

Mwebe, H. (2023). Giving evidence before the First-tier Tribunal (Mental Health): what is the role of inpatient nurses? A review of literature. *British Journal of Mental Health Nursing.* 12(4): pp. 1–4. https://doi.org/10.12968/bjmh.2023.0012 www.magonlinelibrary.com/doi/abs/10.12968/ bjmh.2023.0012

NHS England. (2023). *The Mental Health Nurse's Handbook.* www.england.nhs.uk/long-read/the-men tal-health-nurses-handbook/ [Accessed 25 August 2024].

Nursing and Midwifery Council. (2018). Future nurse: standards of proficiency of registered nurses. www. nmc.org.uk/globalassets/sitedocuments/education-standards/future-nurse-proficiencies.pdf   [Accessed 23 September 2024].

Nursing and Midwifery Council. (2018). *The Code.* The Code: Professional standards of practice and behaviour for nurses, midwives and nursing associates – The Nursing and Midwifery Council. www. nmc.org.uk/standards/code/ [Accessed 23 September 2024].

Pearson, M., and Pringle, A. (2014). Medicines management. In: Callaghan, P., Dickinson, T., and Felton, A. (eds.) *Mental Health Nursing Skills 2e.* Oxford: Oxford University Press.

Public Health England. (2017). *Better Care for People with Co-Occurring Mental Health and Alcohol/ Drug Use Conditions. A Guide for Commissioners and Service Providers.* https://assets.publishing.serv ice.gov.uk/media/5a75b781ed915d6faf2b5276/Co-occurring_mental_health_and_alcohol_drug_use_ conditions.pdf [Accessed 23 September 2024].

Rees, H. (2023). First-tier Tribunal (Mental Health) hearings: protecting the therapeutic relationship. *Nursing Standard.* doi: 10.7748/mhp.2023.e1664

Royal College of Psychiatrists. (2017). *Good Psychiatric Practice: Confidentiality and Information Sharing* (2nd ed.). www.rcpsych.ac.uk/improving-care/campaigning-for-better-mental-health-policy/ college-reports/2017-college-reports/good-psychiatric-practice-confidentiality-and-information-shar ing-2nd-edition-cr209-nov-2017 [Accessed 20 September 2024].

Royal College of Psychiatrists and Tribunals Judiciary. (2017*). A Guide for Trainees: Attending a Mental Health Tribunal Hearing.* www.rcpsych.ac.uk/docs/default-source/training/curricula-and-guidance/ a-guide-for-trainees-observing-tribunals-updated-sept-2019.pdf?sfvrsn=a62a3404_2   [Accessed   23 September 2024].

Soltan, M. (2017). How to approach the mental state examination. *British Medical Journal.* 375. doi: https:// doi.org/10.1136/sbmj.j1821

Teasdale, S., B., Ward, P., B., Rosenbaum, S., Samaras, H., and Stubbs, B. (2017). Solving a weighty problem: systematic review and meta-analysis of nutrition interventions in severe mental illness. *British Journal of Psychiatry.* 210: pp. 110–118.

Ungar, M., and Theron, L. (2020). Resilience and mental health: how multisystemic process contribute to positive outcomes. *The Lancet Psychiatry.* 7(5): pp. 441–448.

Warrender, D., and Young, C. (2024). Considering and responding to risk when working with people living with mental health problems. In: Callaghan, P., Dickinson, T., and Felton, A. (eds.) *Mental Health Nursing Skills 2e*. Oxford: Oxford University Press.

Wood, J., McLaughlin, N.,   and Owen, W. (2017). The person experiencing schizophrenia. Chapter 24. In: Chambers, M. (ed.). *Psychiatric and mental health nursing. The Craft of Caring*. London: Routledge.

11 The Responsible Clinician's Evidence

Gareth Rees

Introduction

As the title of their role suggests, responsible clinicians have an obligation to protect the rights of people experiencing mental distress by ensuring that those liable to detention in hospital (or subject to community treatment orders or guardianship) continue to meet the legal tests (statutory criteria) as set out by the Mental Health Act 1983, amended 2007 (hereafter referred to as *the Act*). One of the ways that responsible clinicians can ensure such patients are treated fairly and in the least restrictive manner is to engage with the safeguards embedded within the Act; the importance of taking an active part in hearings of the First Tier Tribunal (hereafter referred to as *mental health tribunals*) is therefore made explicit in the tribunal rules (Tribunal Procedure Committee, 2008). Whilst mental health tribunals are generally conducted in a more flexible and informal manner than other areas of the judiciary (Hale, 2017), responsible clinicians commonly have very little, if any, formal training regarding tribunal etiquette or giving evidence in legal proceedings (Nimmagadda and Jones, 2008). Navigating the complexities of mental health tribunals can therefore be a daunting experience for them and potentially impact negatively upon their therapeutic relationship with patients (Akther *et al.*, 2019; Macgregor, Brown and Stavert, 2019; Rees, 2023). This chapter aims to remedy this by suggesting a framework for responsible clinicians to use when preparing to give written and oral evidence to the First Tier Tribunal (mental health).

What is a Responsible Clinician?

The 2007 amendments to the Mental Health Act 1983 replaced the position of Responsible Medical Officer (RMO) with two new roles: Responsible Clinician and Approved Clinician (NHS England, 2024). Responsible clinicians are appointed by responsible authorities and can be defined as *approved clinicians with overall responsibility for the patient's care.* They typically come from a medical background (usually psychiatrists) but experienced clinicians from other disciplines (e.g. nursing, psychology, social work) can also now be approved by the secretary of state (NHS England, 2024). The role is particularly relevant for patients liable to detention/supervised community treatment under the Act as some decisions (e.g., issuing Section 17 leave or placing a patient on a Community Treatment Order) can only be made with responsible clinician approval. Other than in some restricted cases (where Home Office approval is necessary), responsible clinicians are also expected to use their authority under Section 23 of the Act to discharge patients who no longer meet the statutory criteria for on-going detention/supervised community treatment/guardianship (Code of Practice, 2015). Given the wide-ranging powers bestowed upon responsible clinicians by the Act, it is unsurprising that Tribunal panels give

DOI: 10.4324/9781003635543-14

their evidence significant weight when making decisions. Indeed, Akther *et al* (2019) argues that Tribunal panels place too much emphasis on the medical model and views of the responsible clinician.

Preparing Written Evidence

Writing reports for mental health tribunals is one of the duties of responsible clinicians and this assists Tribunal panels to reach decisions about patients subject to the conditions of the Act (Care Quality Commission, 2018). Well-written responsible clinician reports (hereafter referred to as *RC reports*) also make hearings less complicated by supporting panels to conduct proceedings safely/efficiently, providing a clear rationale for the responsible authority's position, and making sense of complex clinical information. Conversely, a poorly written RC report reflects badly upon the responsible clinician, distracts from important information, and calls into question the reliability of their evidence. It benefits no one for a hearing to be adjourned because the RC report is determined by the Tribunal panel to be inadequate.

Submitting on Time

In order to give Tribunal panels and patients (in conjunction with their legal representative) sufficient time to consider the written evidence, responsible clinicians have a statutory duty to submit their report in advance of a hearing. The time limits for this are set out in the practice direction issued by Senior President of Tribunals (2013): in all inpatient cases, except where the patient is detained under Section 2 of the Act, the responsible authority must send the required documentation to the Tribunal (and Ministry of Justice for restricted cases) within 3 weeks of receiving the patient's application or reference. Where the patient is detained under Section 2 of the Act, the responsible authority must submit the required documents as soon as is practicable.

Since compiling an RC report can be time-consuming (especially for patients with a long and/ or complex psychiatric history), responsible clinicians should ensure that they set aside sufficient time and resources to complete this task. Indeed, failure to submit on time may result in the Tribunal issuing further directions or imposing sanctions and costs on the responsible authority (Hinchliffe, 2015). Late submissions can also impact on the other professional witnesses, since updated reports may be required if the case is adjourned. It is, therefore, essential that responsible clinicians contact the Tribunal as soon as possible (to request an extension) if there are legitimate reasons as to why they are unable to submit an RC report on time.

Delegation

There may be circumstances in which responsible clinicians need to delegate their duty to prepare an RC report to another clinician e.g., because of sickness/annual leave. Responsible clinicians can also support junior colleagues to meet their educational objectives by allowing them to prepare written evidence on their behalf: the Royal College of Psychiatrists (2019), for example, considers it essential that experienced psychiatry trainees gain experience in report writing so that they can apply to become approved clinicians at the end of their training. However, when responsible clinicians delegate their duty to submit an RC report to the Tribunal, the Code of Practice (2015) is clear that nominated authors need to have *personally met the patient and be familiar with their history and recent presentation*. Nominated authors also need access to appropriate levels of support/supervision, depending on their level of experience writing reports and the complexity of the case. Foundation Year 1 doctors should not be asked to prepare RC reports since they are not fully registered medical practitioners with the General Medical Council (Royal College of Psychiatrists, 2019). All RC reports written by a nominated author must be signed and countersigned by the patient's responsible clinician.

Accessibility

In order to make sure that the Tribunal panel receives complete and up-to-date reports, responsible clinicians should ensure that their written evidence is dated and has numbered pages/paragraphs (Senior President of Tribunals, 2013). Doing so will makes it easier for responsible clinicians to refer to their report and/or be directed to specific parts of their evidence during a Tribunal hearing. RC reports should be made easily accessible to readers by using a clear/consistent font, adequate line spacing, and presenting historical information in chronological order wherever possible. Responsible clinicians should also proofread their reports (to ensure accuracy and avoid spelling/grammar mistakes) and refrain from using unnecessary medical terminology/jargon where possible. As with all other forms of documentation, the possibility of misunderstandings can be reduced by making sure that any abbreviations or acronyms are explained in full (Rees, 2013). It is also considered good practice for responsible clinicians (if safe to do so) to offer their patients an opportunity to read through/discuss the RC report before submission, since inaccurate and/or non-evidence-based information can hinder tribunal proceedings. Doing this also allows responsible clinicians to validate their patient's feelings by addressing/documenting differences of opinion and taking appropriate measures to mitigate potential damage to the therapeutic alliance (Rees, 2023).

If specific information is unavailable at the time of submitting an RC report, it can be added by way of an addendum so long as this is made available to the tribunal panel (and the patient's representative) at least one hour before the hearing is scheduled to begin. Likewise, the Tribunal Procedure Committee (2008) states that if an RC report is outdated, inaccurate or the status of the patient changes before the Tribunal hearing takes place, responsible clinicians should assist the Tribunal by preparing an addendum report addressing any significant updates or amendments.

Non-disclosure

Although patients generally have a right to know why they are detained (Zigmond and Brindle, 2022), Rule 14 of the tribunal rules (Tribunal Procedure Committee, 2008), allows panels to prohibit the disclosure of specific information to a patient if *a) such disclosure would be likely to cause that person or some other person serious harm* and *b) the tribunal is satisfied, having regard to the interests of justice, that it is proportionate to give such a direction.* If a responsible clinician wants the Tribunal panel to consider using this power, they should detail the information they wish to be non-disclosed in a separate document along with full written reasons for their request. This document should also be clearly marked: NOT TO BE DISCLOSED TO THE PATIENT WITHOUT THE EXPRESS PERMISSION OF THE TRIBUNAL. The patient's legal representative is not automatically given a copy of such submissions; however, the Tribunal panel may decide to share it with them if they believe it to be in the interest of the patient. The panel subsequently decides whether the grounds for non-disclosure have been met and conducts the hearing accordingly. Responsible clinicians should therefore be prepared for the possibility that their request is declined and consider contingencies to safeguard their patient (and others) should this occur.

Contents of the RC Report

The practice direction issued by the Senior President of Tribunals in 2013 is legally binding and requires RC reports to contain specific information, depending on whether the patient is an inpatient, community patient, or conditionally discharged. This information assists the Tribunal by identifying factors that may affect the patient's understanding or ability to cope with a hearing (so that the case can be dealt with fairly) as well as addressing the statutory criteria of the Act relevant to the patient being discussed. To make report writing more straightforward for responsible clinicians, responsible authorities often have their own templates based on this practice direction and it is advisable to utilise these if available.

One of the challenges for authors of Tribunal reports is including sufficient information to assist the panel without damaging their therapeutic alliance with the patient (Rees, 2023). Good RC reports are therefore succinct, non-judgmental, and provide specific examples/evidence to justify the author's opinions. As discussed earlier, it is also a good idea for responsible clinicians, if safe to do so, to allow patients to read their RC reports before submission so that any disagreements can be discussed/validated/documented. Whilst it may be tempting to copy and paste information from other documents, the practice direction (2013) is clear that RC reports need to be prepared specifically for the hearing to avoid them containing insufficient, superfluous or out-of-date information. For the same reasons, responsible clinicians should avoid reproducing information from the patient's medical records, unless it is objective and pertinent to the case.

Facilitating the Hearing

As already stated, RC reports need to identify *any factors that may affect the patient's understanding or ability to cope with a hearing* (Tribunal Procedure Committee, 2020). Responsible clinicians are usually well placed to provide this information since they have overall responsibility for the patient's wellbeing and make similar considerations when conducting ward reviews/outpatient clinics, etc. Examples of factors which may be relevant to the Tribunal include communication barriers, impairment of mental capacity and potential triggers for aggression. Being aware of such variables allows Tribunal panels to consider the need to make reasonable adjustments to proceedings in order to facilitate the patient's participation and/or keep other participants safe. Indeed, under Rule 2(4) of the tribunal rules (Tribunal Procedure Committee, 2008), responsible clinicians have a duty to inform the Tribunal if anyone due to attend a hearing could endanger the safety of others and provide information about how these risks might be managed.

Addressing the Statutory Criteria

To assist Tribunal panels in reaching informed and objective decisions about patients liable to detention/supervised community treatment under the Act, the burden of proof is on responsible clinicians to demonstrate in their reports that, on the balance of probabilities, the statutory criteria being relied upon are still met (Brown *et al.*, 2023).

First and foremost, responsible clinicians need to demonstrate that the patient has a mental disorder, defined by the Act as *any disorder or disability of the mind* (MHA, 1983). Whilst this may sound axiomatic, failure to do so contravenes Article 5 of the European Convention of Human Rights (Right to Liberty and security) which only permits, under certain circumstances, people with *unsound mind* from being detained for treatment (Schabas, 2017). Conditions which could fall within the Act's broad definition of mental disorder include, but are not limited to, organic disorders e.g. dementia, affective/mood disorders e.g. depression, psychotic disorders e.g. schizophrenia, neurotic disorders e.g. obsessive-compulsive disorder, eating disorders e.g. anorexia nervosa, and personality disorders. However, according to the Code of Practice (2015), learning disabilities *share few features with the serious mental illnesses that are the most common reason for using the Act* and therefore do not meet the definition unless they are *associated with abnormally aggressive or seriously irresponsible conduct.* Likewise, Section 1(3) of the Act states that dependence on alcohol or drugs must not be used *per se* to justify compulsion.

In order to demonstrate the presence of a mental disorder, responsible clinicians should document the patient's psychiatric diagnoses (which meet the definition of mental disorder) and comorbidities in the RC report. It is important, however, that responsible clinicians avoid diagnosing mental disorders based on preconceptions about a person's cultural/social differences since beliefs/behaviours which are not part of a mental disorder should never be used to justify use of the Act, even when they are unusual or cause distress (Hale, 2017).

When a definitive diagnosis has yet to be made (particularly in Section 2 cases), responsible clinicians can evidence the likely presence of a mental disorder by providing a narrative account of the patient's history, symptomatology and mental state examination. If this is not based on the author's own observations, the RC report should also document which sources of information have been considered to form this view. After evidencing the presence of a mental disorder, RC reports need to describe whether it is the *nature* and/or *degree* of this that makes the patient liable to detention/supervised community treatment. These two terms should be construed distinctly since case law has established that the nature of a patient's mental disorder may make hospital treatment may be appropriate, even when the degree does not – see *R v Mental Health Review Tribunal for the South Thames Region ex p. Smith* (1999). The *nature* of a mental disorder refers to its *chronicity, prognosis, and the patient's previous response to receiving treatment for the disorder*; psychotic disorders, for example, may be short and self-limiting (e.g. in some cases of drug intoxication), or chronic and treatment-resistant (e.g. in some cases of schizophrenia). This information is relevant when deciding upon the appropriateness of compulsion but may only be known for patients who have had previous involvement with mental health services; responsible clinicians should therefore make it clear in the RC report if historical sources of information have been used to ascertain the nature of the patient's mental disorder.

In contrast, the *degree* of a mental disorder refers to its current manifestation and includes the presence/absence/intensity of specific psychiatric symptoms and their impact on the patient's wellbeing/functioning at the time of writing the report. Responsible clinicians should therefore be able to describe the degree of a mental disorder, even if this is the patient's first contact with mental health services. When documenting the degree of a mental disorder, responsible clinicians also need to consider other dynamic factors such as the patient's insight and concordance with treatment. As already stated, it is important that the RC report documents any additional sources of information that have been used. In simple terms, *nature* refers to the type of mental disorder a patient has, whereas *degree* refers to its current severity.

In order for a person to have ongoing liability to detention/supervised community treatment under the Act, there must be an element of risk to the patient or others (Hale, 2017). For the so-called civil sections of the Act, this relates to risks involving the patient's own health, or safety, or the protection of others (with any one of these, or a combination, being acceptable). RC reports therefore need to include a description of the patient's risks and why they are sufficient to justify on-going use of the Act. This can be achieved by summarising the patient's historical, current, and future risks, as well as any mitigating or protective factors. As with documenting the presence of a mental disorder, responsible clinicians may wish to describe these in terms of *nature* and *degree*. They should also provide evidence/examples to justify their opinions and link any risks to the patient's mental disorder. In the case of *R (on the application of LI) v Mental Health Review Tribunal (2004)*, it was held that risks unconnected with the patient's mental disorder were irrelevant to the Tribunal's decision.

The MHA Code of Practice (2015), takes a broad approach to risk; risks to the patient's health, for example, applies to both their physical and mental wellbeing e.g. the risk of self-neglect, stopping treatment for a mental/physical condition, reduced food/fluid intake, relapse. Likewise, when documenting risks to safety, RC reports should consider the patient's acts or omissions e.g. deliberate self-harm and completed suicide, as well as those by others e.g. vulnerability and risk retaliation. Risks pertaining to the protection of others are usually more self-evident and include verbal/physical aggression, violence, disinhibition, and reckless behaviour.

In all compulsory admissions for treatment, both civil and forensic, the 2007 amendments to the Act require *appropriate medical treatment* to be available to the patient (replacing the previously controversial criterion that the patient's mental disorder be *treatable*) (Hale, 2017). However, since the Act defines medical treatment so broadly i.e. anything with positively improves the patient's condition or at least prevents it getting worse, responsible clinicians usually have no problems evidencing this in their reports by documenting what treatment the patient is currently receiving (or has available to them). This includes psychological and social interventions as well as pharmacological treatments such as medication; indeed, in *R v Mersey Mental Health Review Tribunal, Ex p. D (1987)*, it was held appropriate to continue compulsory treatment for a patient who was only able to access basic nursing care.

Depending on which section(s) of the Act are being used, RC reports need to include other specific information. In the case of inpatients, for example, RC reports should document whether any risks could be managed effectively in the community (and how). Conversely, RC reports for patients subject to supervised community treatment need to describe why the power of hospital recall remains necessary, and whether the patient is compliant with the conditions of their community treatment order. The practice direction (2013), is very clear about what information needs to be included in the RC report depending on whether the patient is an inpatient or subject to supervised community treatment, guardianship or conditional discharge. If a responsible clinician is unsure about this, it would therefore be advisable to use a template based on the practice direction and/or seek advice from a mental health act administrator.

Other Considerations

Regardless of whether the patient is detained in hospital or subject to guardianship/supervised community treatment/conditional discharge, all RC reports need to provide a summary of the patient's current progress, behaviour, capacity and insight (Senior President of Tribunals, 2013). This information allows the panel to form an impression about the patient's recovery and whether or not there is a possibility that they could be managed in a less restrictive setting. Responsible clinicians who know their patients well are unlikely to have difficulty in articulating these opinions. In order for Tribunal panels to consider whether the patient could be managed informally/voluntarily, RC reports should also describe what treatment would be available to the patient if they were no longer subject to compulsion under the Act, and whether they would have mental capacity to agree/decline this. Although mental capacity is not referred to in the statutory criteria of the Act, Tribunal panels are likely to be interested in whether the patient can provide capacious consent to treatment when coming to a decision about the need for compulsion. When commenting on a patient's mental capacity, responsible clinicians should also remember to abide by the principles of the Mental Capacity Act (2005), i.e. presumption of capacity, supporting patients to make their own decisions, accepting unwise decisions, considering best interests, and promoting least restrictive options.

As already alluded to in this chapter, patients liable to detention/supervised community treatment under the Act can find information about their symptoms and risks distressing to read (Macgregor, Brown and Stavert, 2019; Rees, 2023). Responsible clinicians should, therefore, attempt to improve this, where possible, by dedicating a section of the RC report to the patient's strengths and positive factors which might help in their recovery. Doing this also encourages Tribunal panels to consider patients in a holistic and recovery-focussed manner. However, responsible clinicians need to ensure that the information included in this section is not deemed by the patient to be patronising or tokenistic, as this may have the opposite of the desired effect.

Finally, at the end of the RC report, the practice direction (2013) advises responsible clinicians to outline their overall recommendation(s) to the Tribunal. This should be clear, concise and evidence-based where possible. Like all legal documents, RC reports need to be signed and dated by the author.

Attending Mental Health Tribunals

Except for automatic referrals of patients subject to Community Treatment Orders where the outcome is agreed, the Tribunal is unable to dispose of proceedings without holding a hearing (Hale, 2017). Although they are generally conducted in a more flexible and informal manner than other court proceedings, mental health tribunals make potentially life-changing decisions about patients liable to detention/compulsory supervised treatment. In keeping with the Code of Practice (2015), there is therefore an expectation that responsible clinicians will attend hearings in person and submit their availability to the Tribunal in advance. If there is a genuine reason why the responsible clinician is unable to attend, they should make the Tribunal aware of this and ask a suitable colleague to attend in their absence. According to guidance produced by the Royal College of Psychiatrists (2019), psychiatry trainees can also give oral evidence on behalf of the responsible clinician provided that:

a) they have supervised experience of writing an RC report,
b) they have observed a hearing and given evidence under supervision of the responsible clinician,
c) the responsible clinician is satisfied that they are competent to give evidence, and
d) the responsible clinician has agreed that it is an appropriate case for them to give evidence.

Remote Hearings

In order to remain compatible with Articles 6 (*Right to Liberty and Security, and Right to a Fair Trial*) and 5(4) (*that detention shall be decided speedily by a court*) of the European Convention of Human Rights (Schabas, 2017), the practice direction issued by the Tribunal Procedure Committee in March 2020 (in response to the Covid pandemic) enabled the First Tier Tribunal (mental health) to start conducting hearings remotely. Since then, mental health patients have retained the right to request remote hearings using the videoconferencing platform procured by the Ministry of Justice (known as CVP).

Procedurally, remote hearings are conducted in almost an identical way to those held in-person. However, in order to prepare for a remote hearing, responsible clinicians need to ensure that they have the correct equipment to join CVP e.g. a working microphone/webcam, supported web browser and stable internet connection. Responsible clinicians should also ensure that their devices have sufficient power to last the entirety of the hearing and that they are aware of the link being used (this will be supplied by the Tribunal in advance). Finally, since most mental health tribunals are held in private (Hale, 2017), responsible clinicians need to ensure that nobody else in the room with them (without the expression permission of the Tribunal) and that they will not be overheard giving evidence; failure to do so may result in responsible clinicians being held in contempt of court.

General Advice

Since mental health tribunals are court proceedings, it is advisable for responsible clinicians to dress smartly and conduct themselves accordingly. Regardless of whether the hearing is to be conducted remotely or in-person, responsible clinicians should also be punctual, and allow time for the panel to discuss any preliminary matters e.g. issues regarding the patient's mental capacity. As previously stated, it is good practice to for responsible clinicians to discuss their RC report with the patient before the hearing (to validate/document any disagreements). It is also advisable for responsible clinicians to read the reports prepared by the other professional witnesses in order to anticipate any differences of opinion. Finally, responsible clinicians should ensure that they have had recent contact with the patient so that they are in a position to provide the panel with up-to-date information about the patient's mental state and risks.

There may be situations when it may be appropriate/beneficial for observers to attend mental health tribunals e.g. solicitors intending to undertake mental health work, clinicians who wish to gain experience of giving evidence, or friends/relatives of the patient wishing to give support (HM Courts and Tribunal Service, 2019). However, if a responsible clinician wishes to invite an observer to the hearing, it is advisable to gain permission from the patient and submit an application to the Tribunal in advance. When making a decision about whether to allow an observer, the Tribunal will apply Rule 2 of the tribunal rules (Tribunal Procedure Committee, 2008) to ensure that all parties are still able to participate fully in proceedings e.g. the request will be rejected if the presence of an observer is likely to cause distress for the patient or intimidate one of the professional witnesses. If their presence is agreed by the panel, it is important that observers must play no part in the hearing and sit somewhere unobtrusive. They are allowed to make notes (so long as they are confidential) but should be reminded that any attempt to record the proceedings, may be considered a contempt of court.

The Hearing Itself

Oral evidence will be taken from the professional witnesses in a systematic fashion once the mental health tribunal has commenced: although the tribunal rules (2008) do not prescribe a set order, responsible clinicians will normally give evidence first by answering questions from Tribunal panel members, and the patient's legal representative. Usually this will begin with a request to provide the Tribunal with an update regarding the patient's progress since the RC report was written. Some judges also like to confirm with the responsible clinician at the outset whether they still believe the statutory criteria of the Act are still met. After this, responsible clinicians should be prepared to clarify and expand upon (if necessary) the information provided to the Tribunal in their written evidence. It is therefore good practice for responsible clinicians to bring a copy of their report to the hearing and familiarise themselves with its contents beforehand.

Responsible clinicians should be succinct and direct their answers to the panel rather than the patient (or their legal representative). They should also speak slowly and clearly so that their evidence is comprehensible, and the Tribunal Judge has an opportunity to document what has been said. Wherever possible, responsible clinicians should provide evidence/specific examples to support their opinions; in order to minimise potential damage to the therapeutic alliance, it is also advisable for their responses to be balanced, patient-centred and recovery-focussed. It is okay for responsible clinicians to say that they do not know the answer to a question or to ask for it to be repeated/rephrased in a different way. Where the facts of the case are disputed, the Tribunal will use the ordinary civil standard of proof i.e. on the balance of probabilities (Hale, 2017).

On request to the panel, responsible clinicians can be given permission to be released from a mental health tribunal after giving oral evidence. However, unless absolutely essential, responsible clinicians should consider staying for the remainder of the hearing. Doing so not only demonstrates professionalism and respect for the patient/legal process, but also means that they are available to offer support the other professional witnesses and monitor the patient's well-being/safety. If it becomes apparent that the patient's risks are escalating, responsible clinicians should inform the Tribunal panel and may be asked to suggest the best way forward and/or of mitigating the risks. If the responsible clinician decides to remain in the hearing after giving evidence, it is also important that they do not challenge any oral evidence provided by the other professional witnesses or offer clarification/comments to the panel unless specifically directed to do so (including after the hearing has concluded).

After the Hearing

Patients are likely to experience a range of emotions after listening to the oral evidence presented by the professional witnesses at a mental health tribunal (Akther *et al.*, 2019). At the end of a hearing, it is therefore essential that the responsible clinician supports the Tribunal panel to identify and mitigate potential escalations of the patient's risk profile. This is particularly relevant when the Tribunal's decision goes against the wishes of the patient and/or in remote hearings where the responsible clinician is less likely to be in the immediate vicinity of the patient when the decision is announced. In some situations it may be necessary for the responsible clinician to meet with the patient immediately after the hearing to discuss the panel's decision and its ramifications.

Regardless of the outcome of a mental health tribunal, responsible clinicians should ensure that the panel's decision is contemporaneously recorded in the patient's care record. This prevents any confusion about the patient's legal status and allows the treating team to make any necessary amendments to the patient's risk assessment and treatment/care plan.

Where appropriate and safe to do so, responsible clinicians should also make time to read and discuss the Tribunal's written decision with the patient when available. This provides an opportunity for reflection, psychoeducation and potential amelioration of any damage to the therapeutic alliance caused by the hearing itself (Rees, 2023).

Conclusion

Participating in mental health tribunals can be a tightrope walk for responsible clinicians, balancing their obligation to provide clear and comprehensive information with their clinical obligation to maintain a therapeutic alliance and protect patients from unnecessary distress. However, responsible clinicians needn't feel daunted by the prospect of giving evidence; to the contrary, by following the framework set out in this chapter, responsible clinicians have an opportunity to champion their patient's rights and support the First Tier Tribunal (mental health) to make fair and evidence-based decisions.

References

Akther, S.F. *et al*. (2019) 'Patients' experiences of assessment and detention under mental health legislation: systematic review and qualitative meta-synthesis'. *BJ Psych Open*, 5: 3.

Brown, R. *et al*. (2023) *Mental Health Law in England and Wales*. SAGE.

Care Quality Commission. (2018) Mental Health Act: Approved Mental Health Professional Services. Available at: www.cqc.org.uk/sites/default/ files/20180326_mha_amhpbriefing.pdf (Accessed: 12 October 2024).

Department of Health and Social Care. (2015) *Mental Health Act 1983: Code of Practice*. The Stationery Office.

Hale, B. (2017) *Mental Health Law*. 6th ed. Sweet and Maxwell.

Hinchliffe, M. (2015) *Failure to Submit Reports to the Tribunal on Time*, 17 April. [Letter]. Available at: www.mentalhealthlaw.co.uk/media/MHT_letter_re_failure_to_submit_reports_to_the_tribunal_on_time_17_Apr_2015.pdf (Accessed: 13 October 2024).

HM Courts and Tribunal Service. (2019) *Guidance for the Observation of Tribunal Hearings*. Available at: https://assets.publishing.service.gov.uk/media/60c761c6e90e0743a8ed36a0/t120-eng.pdf (Accessed: 15 October 2024).

Macgregor, A., Brown, M., and Stavert, J. (2019) 'Are mental health tribunals operating in accordance with international human rights standards? A systematic review of the international literature'. *Health and Social Care in the Community*, 27: 4.

MHA (1983) (amended 2007) Mental Health Act. Department of Health, London, The Stationery Office.

NHS England. (2024) *Approved Clinicians and Responsible Clinicians (AC/RC)*. Available at: www.hee.nhs.uk/our-work/mental-health/new-ways-working-mental-health/approved-clinicians-responsible-clinicians-acrc (Accessed: 13 October 2024).

Nimmagadda, S., and Jones, C.N. (2008) 'Consultant psychiatrists' knowledge of their role as representatives of the responsible authority at mental health review tribunals'. *Psychiatric Bulletin*, 32: 366–9.

Rees, G. (2013) 'Staff use of acronyms in electronic care records'. *Mental Health Practice*, 16(10): 28–31.

Rees, H. (2023) 'First-tier Tribunal (Mental Health) hearings: protecting the therapeutic relationship'. *Mental Health Practice*, 26(6): 35–42.

Royal College of Psychiatrists. (2019) *Guidance for Detaining Authorities and Tribunal Panels and Medical Evidence of First Tier Tribunal Mental Health*. Available at: www.rcpsych.ac.uk/docs/default-source/training/curricula-and-guidance/guidance-for-detaining-authorities-and-tribunal-panels-about-medical-evidence-for-first-tier-tribunal-may-2019-for-college-comments.docx?sfvrsn=295d0f52_2 (Accessed: 12 October 2024).

Schabas, W.A. (2017) *The European Convention on Human Rights*. Oxford University Press.

Senior President of Tribunals. (2013) *Statement and Reports in Mental Health Cases*. Available at: www.mentalhealthlaw.co.uk/media/Practice_Direction_on_Reports_28_Oct_2013.pdf (Accessed: 12 October 2024).

Tribunal Procedure Committee. (2008) *Health Education and Social Care Chamber Tribunal Rules*. Available at: www.gov.uk/government/publications/health-education-and-social-care-chamber-tribunal-rules (Accessed: 12 October 2024).

Tribunal Procedure Committee. (2020) *The Tribunal Procedure (Coronavirus) (Amendment) Rules*. Available at: www.gov.uk/government/publications/tribunal-procedure-committee-rules (Accessed: 12 October 2024).

Zigmond, T., and Brindle, N. (2022) *A Clinician's Brief Guide to the Mental Health Act*. 5th ed. Cambridge University Press.

Case Law

R (on the application of LI) v Mental Health Review Tribunal (2004).
R v Mental Health Review Tribunal for the South Thames Region ex p. Smith (1999).
R v Mersey Mental Health Review Tribunal, Ex p. D (1987).

12 The Care Coordinator's Evidence

Ruairi Mulhern and Lorraine Summers

Introduction – Social Circumstance Reports

In this chapter the term "patient" is used to denote a mental health service user that is subject to the coercive powers of the Mental Health Act, either in a hospital or in the community. Patient is routinely used in legislation and associated documentation, including pro forma social circumstance report documents. For some people, the term has negative connotations not least due to the implicit suggestion that the patient is a passive recipient of care from an expert. This view is contested within mental health survivor networks, and it could be argued that it is a term that is, perhaps, more suited to physical health care. However it is important to acknowledge that the discussion about which term is the most appropriate to use is complicated. For example, in an exploration of the appropriate term to use Priebe (2021), argued that: "The term 'service user' in this context should be avoided.........: the term is discriminating, cynical, patronising and detrimental. Of course, none of these effects is intentional, but that does not change them", (Priebe, 2021, p.327).
    According to Priebe (2021)

> The term 'patient', however, describes appropriately a temporary role in healthcare, provides parity of esteem with patients in physical healthcare, and reflects the reasons why large parts of society are willing to fund healthcare, in solidarity with those who are sick.
>
> (Priebe, 2021)

It was further observed that:

> A number of surveys have asked patients in mental health services which term they prefer to be used. The results of these surveys are consistent. The majority of patients prefer the term patient, and this applies across studies that have been conducted at different times and in different settings.
>
> (Priebe, 2021, p.328)

Social circumstances reports are a routine duty for any mental health professional working in hospital or in secondary care, most typically in a community mental health service. It is envisaged that the incoming Mental Health Act (2025) the demand for these reports is likely to increase. The social circumstance reports are, in essence, no different from other reports that are produced by professional staff. As expected in different forums, professional staff are required to produce and speak to assessment reports, case summaries, and discharge summaries. These reports and summaries are in effect a professionals account of a patient's circumstance

DOI: 10.4324/9781003635543-15

(condition) and situation (what has or is happening). The aim of any such reports is to provide other professionals with the necessary information that would enable them to have a better understanding of what is happening and, as appropriate, how to proceed. For example, the Hospital Mangers Hearing is a review process where a panel of independent individuals, known as hospital managers, assess whether a patient should continue to be detained under the Act. Similar to First Tier Tribunal the managers hearing panel will review reports, including a social circumstances report, and have the authority to discharge patients from detention. However, the hearing is not a legal court, and the panel are not legal or medical experts, so they tend to be less formal than a tribunal. Managers hearings typically occur when a detained patient, including someone subject to a Community Treatment Order (CTO) does not exercise their right to appeal their detention to the tribunal.

The manager's hearing is a safeguard to ensure that the authority for detaining a patient is in order and any relevant documents are correct. Chapter 37 of the Code Of Practice to the Mental Health Act (1983) details the functions of hospital managers, (Department of Health and Social Care, 2015). A social circumstances report submitted to a managers' hearing should be to the same standard as a report for the tribunal, but it is possible that you will not be required at a physical hearing as managers hearing can in certain circumstances review the documents without a physical meeting. Section 68 of the Mental Health Act 1983 outlines the duties of hospital managers to refer certain patients' cases to a tribunal. This section ensures that patients who do not exercise their rights to apply to a tribunal are still provided with judicial oversight.

Legal Obligation to First Tier Tribunal

In contrast to the Manager's Hearing and the provision of other reports for the different forums, the request to prepare a social circumstances report may come from a Mental Health Act Administrator, usually an NHS Trust employee, on behalf of the Mental Health Tribunal, formally referred to as the First-tier Tribunal. The tribunal is considered a court within the UK judicial system and the reports are statutory requirements that must meet certain rules regarding content and timing. Tribunals are not hospital meetings, and the reports presented are not staff handovers. They are formal documents and must withstand legal scrutiny. Any staff writing a report must be clear about the statutory requirements they face and the powers of the tribunal. It is important to treat the request to produce a report as a priority, team managers should know this, and your Mental Health Act office will certainly support this position.

At its core, a tribunal hearing will decide on the liberty of a fellow citizen, so it is crucial that all efforts are both professional and person centred. Hence the requirement that health and social care professionals fulfil this task as perfectly suited to the roll. Reports will be examined by the tribunal panel but also the service users and their legal representative so objective evidence-based conclusions and recommendations need to be rational and clear. You will attend the tribunal and address any questions based on your written report. There are occasions when the report writer is not the person giving evidence, in such circumstance it is crucial that whoever is giving evidence has taken the time to not only read the report that they will be presenting but also show professional curiosity about the case. This means finding out any additional information that may be of interest or concern to the panel. The tribunal, as it is required and directed by the Senior President of Tribunals, would expect:

> The report must be up-to-date, specifically prepared for the tribunal, and have numbered paragraphs and pages. It should be signed and dated. The sources of information for the events and incidents described must be made clear. This report should not be an addendum to

(or reproduce extensive details from) previous reports, but must briefly describe the patient's recent relevant history and current presentation. ...

(Sullivan, J, 2013, p.4)

Who Completes the Report?

There is no specific stipulation as to which professional is responsible for completing the report only that they "should have personally met and be familiar with the patient", (Practice Direction, 2013). In practice a report is most likely to be completed by either the community mental health nurse, social worker, or occupational therapist. Having an approved mental health professional qualification would be an advantage but is not a requirement. In recent years, many community mental health services have recruited talented and experienced non-professional community staff who act as key workers or de facto care coordinators as part of the Community Mental Health Framework. They can be an asset in completing a report, but the author must be a professional member of staff. The pro forma specifically requests the "views of any other person who takes a lead role in the care and support of the patient but who is not professionally involved". It's also possible that the patient is new to mental health services and does not have statutory community support, professional or otherwise. In such cases, it's for the professional completing the report to become familiar, meeting the patient, relevant others, including nearest relative/nominated person and reviewing documentation. Familiarity with a patient does not hinge on an established therapeutic relationship.

Pro Forma Documents Inpatient or Community Report?

Standardised documents that meet the requirements for social circumstances reporting are available from the Gov.UK website along with all other official pro forma required under mental health legislation, and more. Social Circumstance reports will be required for either an inpatient or a community patient but as the Mental Health Act has no age limits the report may be required for a child as well as an adult, (GOV.UK, n.d.).

Form T133: In-patient: Social Circumstances Report for In-patients

A request to complete a Social Circumstances Report will most likely be in relation to an "in-patient" detained under section two or three of the Mental Health Act (1983). Generally, a significant majority of tribunals are for in-patients, as they are more frequently subject to compulsory treatment under the Mental Health Act. For example, in 2021-2022, around 80 per cent of tribunal hearings were for in-patients, (CQC, 2022).

Form T138 is Used to Create a Social Circumstances Report for Community Patients

This report provides detailed information about the patient's social background, living conditions, and support network, similar to that required for the 'in-patient' report. The majority of such reports deal with Community Treatment Orders (CTO) however they also cover the small number (115 in 2021) of patient's subject to Guardianship (section 7 MHA). Around 20 per cent of tribunal hearings are for community patients, (CQC, 2022). About 5500 patients are subject to CTOs at any one time. The low rate of CTO discharges by mental health tribunals (below 5%) suggests that they are not used inappropriately, (Gupta et al., 2018).

Form T135: Social circumstances report: Supplementary information required for patients under the age of 18 [B]: In the 2022-23 period, there were 997 detentions recorded for children and young people, with a significant portion of these being aged 16 or 17, (NHS Digital, 2022).

Principles, Policy and Practice in Writing a Social Circumstances Report

Principles: The Mental Health Bill (2025) includes four core principles outlined in the Wessely et al independent review of the 1983 Act (2019). These are;

- Choice and autonomy
- Least restriction
- Therapeutic benefit
- Treating the person as an individual.

Principles can at times seem abstract when faced with the demand to complete a social circumstances report on a person you may not know and at a time when you are already under competing work pressures. A risk is that the completion of a social circumstances report becomes a perfunctory task that lacks professional curiosity, sensitivity, and understanding. It is worth reminding ourselves of the values and principles that underpin our support for a fellow citizen, especially one subject to the coercive powers of the mental health act. Health and social care professionals are duty bound by codes of professional practice to be non-judgemental, honest, and prioritise the service user, (NMC, 2024; SWE, 2019). This is not to say that we will always agree with their requests, but any decision we reach regarding them and their care must be unbiased, clear, and in their best interests. This is not to say that staff never make mistakes, but we must never be motivated by the "needs of the service" or unduly influenced out of a distorted sense of deference to other, possibly more senior colleagues.

The quality of a social circumstances report must be high and the potential consequences for the patient involved central in all thinking and actions. Putting principles into action can have major consequences on occasion. If a nearest relative or nominated person is contacted regarding a social circumstances' report it can be an opportunity to review their knowledge of their rights or powers in that role. Specifically, the nominated person can request the discharge from section of the patient. Under section 23 the nearest relative or nominated person has the power to "order" discharge from section two or section three or CTO; however, this right is qualified by the provisions of section 25, (MHA, 1983). The request must be in writing and the hospital or detaining authority has 72 hours in which to bar the request "if they believe it would be dangerous to discharge" or not. The risk criteria in relation to "dangerousness" is higher than that required to purely detain someone under the act, (MHA, 1983). The NR must give the hospital managers 72 hours' notice of his intention to discharge the patient. They can use a form or write a letter. The Illustrative standard letter for nearest relatives to use to discharge patients can be found in the MHA Code of Practice, para 35.25:

Practice

Social circumstances reports can be influential and deal with issues of principle but in practical terms a reports content must be clear and concise, accurate and relevant. The social circumstances report will, in most instances, be considered in collaboration with a nurse's report and a medical report. Its remit is essentially to provide detailed information about a patient's social background, including their living situation, family relationships, and social support network. This information helps tribunals and hospital managers make informed decisions about the patient's care and potential discharge.

Gathering Information

Access previous records. You may need to request electronic records from several electronic record systems, for example RiO, CareNotes, Digital Social Care Records etc,, so plan ahead and recruit the aid of your Trust or Local Authorities information governance team to assist. It is possible that paper records may be retrieved from Iron Mountain so allow time and seek help via management on how to access old records. Work closely with other professionals involved in the patient's care to ensure all relevant information is included. Best practice recommendations emphasize the importance of collaboration with other professionals, regular updates to the report, and the inclusion of the patient's voice and preferences. These practices help ensure that the report is a holistic and accurate reflection of the patient's social circumstances. Central must be the voice of the patient so where possible include quotes particularly if there is point of contention. Likewise, with family members, nominated person and nearest relative and others who provide care but are not professionally involved use quotes and clarify with them that you will use their quotes in the report to ensure their message is clear and their views communicated.

Social Circumstances Reports – Four Key Areas

1. Informing Decisions

Social circumstances reports provide detailed information about a patient's social background. Collect detailed information about the patient's living situation, support network, employment status, financial situation, and any legal issues. The panel need to know if discharged what housing or accommodation would be available to the patient? Do they have their own secure tenancy or is this in jeopardy due to admission to hospital, for example, if private renting and unable to make payments? Is their accommodation in fit condition to be lived in? If friends or family are in a position to offer a place to stay and if so for how long? An understanding of the home and family circumstances will be necessary if indeed they have such a support network. Understanding who they have or could go to in a financial or housing crisis will help identify resources they have but may not have previously used. It would be incumbent on the staff member to follow this up and record the veracity of the information. For patients who may be recently arrived in the country social networks may be less visible to staff but still exist. Contact with family that are oversees may require engaging the interpreting services, however the result may be a revelation in terms of support hitherto unknown to staff. Staff are not required to be detectives, but a reasonable degree of professional curiosity is demanded given the fact that a person's liberty may be involved. The patient's financial position (including benefit entitlements) and any available opportunities for employment will also be required,

2. Assessing Needs

The reports assess the social care and support needs of the patient, identifying what services and support would be necessary if the patient were to be discharged into the community. This will require an understanding of historic and current care issues including details of any index offence(s), and other relevant forensic history. A chronology listing the patient's previous involvement with mental health services including any admissions to, discharge from, and recall to hospital needs to be included. There needs to be summary provided of the patient's current progress, behaviour, compliance, and insight. Details of any incidents where the patient has harmed themselves or others, or threatened harm, or damaged property, or threatened damage would also need to be added. Is the patient known to any Multi Agency Public Protection Agency, MAPPA meeting or agency and, if so, in which area, for what reason, and at what level-together with the name of the Chair of any MAPPA meeting concerned with the patient, and the name of the representative of the lead agency. In the event that a MAPPA meeting or agency wishes to put forward evidence of its views in relation to the level and management of risk, a summary of those views (or an Executive Summary) may be attached to the report and where ever it is relevant. A copy of the Police National Computer record of previous convictions should be attached. In the case of an eligible compliant patient who lacks capacity to agree or object to their detention or treatment, decisions on whether or not a deprivation of liberty under the Mental Capacity Act 2005 (as amended) would be appropriate and less restrictive would need to be made. There would also need to be a decision on whether (in Section 2 cases) detention in hospital, or (in all other cases) the provision of medical treatment in hospital, is justified or necessary in the interests of the patient's health or safety, or for the protection of others. Would the patient, if discharged from hospital, be likely to act in a manner dangerous to themselves or to others, and if so how, are there any risks that could be managed effectively in the community, including the use of any lawful conditions or recall powers, (Naik, 2017).

3. Planning Aftercare

Reports are crucial for planning aftercare services under Section 117 of the Mental Health Act. They outline the coordination between various public bodies and the specific aftercare arrangements that will be put in place. There would need to be consideration on how well has the patient's previous response to community support or Section 117 aftercare had been received and conducted. So far as is known, details of the care pathway and Section 117 aftercare have to be made available to the patient, together with details of the proposed care plan. What is the likelihood that the proposed care plan would be adequate and effective, and would there be any issues funding the proposed care plan and, if so, what date would these issues will be resolved. The strengths or positive factors relating to the patient should be listed along with the patient's views, wishes, beliefs, opinions, hopes, and concerns, (Naik, 2017; Curran, Golightley and Fennell, 2010).

4. Legal Requirements

Completing a report is a statutory requirement whenever requested by a mental health administrator. This ensures that all relevant social factors are considered in the patient's care plan. If there are any factors that might affect the patient's understanding or ability to cope with a hearing, would there be any adjustments that the tribunal may consider in order to deal with the case fairly and justly? These must be made known to the panel. Any recommendations to the tribunal, with reasons should be submitted. The Mental Health Act Code of Practice (2015) provides detailed guidance on the preparation of reports. It outlines the essential components of the report, including the patient's current social circumstances, historical context, and professional assessments. These are also clear in the pro forma documentation, however:

It is a matter of personal preference whether the report goes further than merely meeting the regulatory requirements.

(Curran, C, Golightley, M and Fennell, P, 2010, p.30)

All reports will be unique and individual so staff should exercise their professional skill and prioritise and detail those parts that have the most bearing on the likelihood of the panel coming to an informed decision. As an adjunct to the legal requirements, local authorities or NHS mental health trusts often have their own specific guidelines for preparing reports. Staff should use these guidelines as an aid to report writing, (Curran, Golightley and Fennell, 2010).

Best Practices Checklist for Preparing Social Circumstances Reports

Reports should be structured appropriately and taking account of relevant and up-to-date guidance. Practitioners should ideally use the pro forma, which is periodically updated, and contains the comprehensive level of information required by the tribunal.

Patient-Centred Approach: This includes the patient's voice, reflecting the patient's views and preferences in the report. This ensures that the patient's perspective is considered in the tribunal's decision-making process.

- *Respect and sensitivity:* Handle sensitive information with care and respect the patient's privacy and dignity.
- *Timeliness and accuracy:* A report should be available up to three weeks prior to tribunal hearing. If significant time has passed since the initial drafting, include an addendum to update the information. Submit your report to the mental health act office and if there is any delay, for any reason, keep them updated.
- Double-check all details for accuracy to avoid any misinformation that could affect the tribunal's decision.
- *Professional Standards:* Adhere to professional standards and ethical guidelines, ensuring confidentiality and integrity in the report.
- *Regulatory Compliance:* Adhere to the Tribunal Procedure Rules and any local authority guidelines. Ensure the report meets all regulatory requirements.
- *Avoid Jargon:* Write in plain language to ensure the report is easily understood by all parties involved.

Common Mistakes in Social Circumstances Reports

1. Recycling old reports / cut and paste: It is important and professional to always draft a new report or thoroughly update an existing one to ensure it accurately reflects the current situation. The gravity of a tribunal hearing demands that staff give the patient and the process the respect that they deserve. It reflects badly on the individual giving evidence and the profession, as a whole, when reports are presented that are not only out of the date, but contained inaccurate, unsubstantiated, and poorly presented information.
2. Lack of Detail: During the hearing, panel members will question witnesses to clarify the information being presented. It is more than likely that the patient's legal representative may challenge the veracity of the evidence being presented. Providing vague, unsupported claims, or insufficient details about the patient's social circumstances is poor practice and will be exposed under cross-questioning.
3. Omitting the patient's voice: Ensure the report reflects the patient's perspective and includes their input wherever possible especially considering the Mental Health Bill (2025), that adding statutory weight to the voice of patients.

4. Failure to Address All Relevant Issues: Ignoring important aspects of the patient's social circumstances that could impact their care and treatment.

5. Inadequate Collaboration: It is good practice, where relevant, to collaborate with healthcare providers, therapists, and other relevant professionals to gather a holistic view of the patient's situation. The motivation must be genuine and related to gathering information and not just evidence that you tried to collaborate. While it is sometimes difficult to get response from other professionals due to unanswered call or emails there is still an expectation by the Tribunal that the Social Circumstances author has exhausted all avenues to seek the necessary information prior to the hearing.

Over-representation – Black Patients' Experience?

The draft Mental Health Bill, (2024), addresses the issue of disproportionate detentions of black people under the Mental Health Act (1983). The bill acknowledges that black people are significantly more likely to be detained under the Mental Health Act compared to white people. For example, Black individuals are 3.5 times more likely to be detained. The bill includes measures aimed at reducing these disparities. This involves improving the cultural competence of mental health services and ensuring that care is more personalized and equitable. There is also an emphasis on enhancing community-based mental health support to prevent unnecessary detentions and provide early intervention, (Joint Committee, 2022). It is reasonable to say that increased scrutiny of social circumstances reports with their attention to community-based care and after care will be one tool to address this long-known injustice.

The disproportion is not limited to detention into hospital alone but also extends to the use of CTO's. In 2021-22 amongst broad ethnic groups also known as the global majority, CTO use was highest for Black or Black British people, (75.5 uses per 100,000 population). This was over 11 times the rate for the White group (6.8 uses per 100,000 population). NHS Digital (2022). Under the new mental health act (2025) existing CTOs will be reviewed under new, stricter criteria to ensure they are still necessary and appropriate, (CQC, 2022). These changes aim to ensure that CTOs are used more appropriately and that patients receive better, more personalized care. The NHS Long Term Plan and the Mental Health Act reforms are closely related, both aiming to improve mental health care in the UK. Both the Long-Term Plan and the Mental Health Act emphasize the importance of community-based care. This includes the Community Mental Health Framework, every person who requires support, care and treatment in the community should have a co-produced and personalised care plan that considers all of their needs, as well as their rights under the Care Act (2016), and Section 117 of the Mental Health Act (1983), when required. This policy landscape dovetails with changes mentioned in the orientation of social circumstances reports. The move toward a more rights-based approach to appreciate people and their circumstances and in particular the disparities faced by the global majority and black service users in particular. The responsibility for addressing and reversing inequalities does not fall alone on the author of social circumstances reports but moving forward the increased attention on culturally informed care should witness a significant growing change.

Mental Health Bill 2025 Tribunal Service Changes

The Mental Health Bill (2025), is a proposed law introduced to Parliament on 6 November, 2024. It is bipartisan with cross party support and expected to become law. The new Mental Health Act 2025 will follow the direction of previous changes with an increased orientation toward a more human rights-based approach to care and treatment. Specific proposals introduce several key changes to the tribunal service to enhance patient rights and streamline processes:

Shortened Detention Periods: The bill proposes shorter initial detention periods before a tribunal review is required, ensuring quicker access to justice for patients.

More Frequent Reviews: There will be more frequent mandatory reviews of detention and treatment decisions, giving patients more opportunities to challenge their status.

Increased Tribunal Hearings: The number of tribunal hearings is expected to increase, and consequentially the number of social circumstances reports.

Nearest Relative change to Nominated Person: A "nominated person" will replace the role of the "nearest relative" and be someone chosen by the patient to represent their interests and support them during their detention. This role is introduced to give patients more control over who advocates for them by removing the potential for detrimental actions by a relative assigned according to section 26 of the 1983 Act, (Wessely et al., 2019). Any general social circumstances report will require the views of the nearest relative or nominated person.

These changes the mental health act aim to improve the fairness and efficiency of the tribunal process, ensuring that patients' rights are better protected.

Conclusion

Newly-qualified staff preparing their first such report should be alerted to the fact they may find reference to redundant terms like Mental Health Review Tribunal or Approved Social Worker online or from older colleagues. This can be confusing so keeping pace with terminology, rules and laws that regulate what we must and must not do is important. A reminder regarding some central aspects of the Mental Health Act (1983). This act of Parliament was amended (updated) in 2007. The Act sets out the rules or legal requirements that govern mental health care in England and Wales, including tribunals. The Act is dense and legalistic whereas the accompanying Code of Practice to the Mental Health Act (1983), designed to explain how the Act should be used, is easily readable and user friendly. The Tribunals, Courts, and Enforcement Act, (2007) is the Act under which Social Circumstances Report was made a regulatory requirement. This act also updated the tribunal service, dispensing with the term Review Tribunal just as the Mental Health Act amendment of 2007 replaced "approved social worker" with "approved mental health professional". Laws are amended or renewed in order to stay relevant within a changing society. Of relevance is the planned Mental Health Act (2025), with the continuing orientation towards a more rights-based approach to care with less coercion and detention, particularly in relation to racial disparities faced by people. By avoiding these common mistakes, reports can be more effective in providing a comprehensive and accurate picture of the patient's social circumstances, ultimately supporting fair, and informed tribunal decisions.

References

Care Act (2016). GOV.UK

CQC (2022) Mental Health Act community treatments orders (CTO) – focused visits report. www.cqc.org.uk/publication/cto-focused-visits/report

Curran, C., Golightley, M., and Fennell, P. (2010) Social circumstances reports for mental health tribunals – part 2. www.mentalhealthlaw.co.uk/media/Legal_Action_-_social_circumstances_reports_part_2_-_July_2010.pdf

Department of Health and Social Care (2015). Code of Practice : Mental Health Act 1983 Online: code of practice: Mental Health Act 1983-GOV.UK

Gov.Uk. (n.d.) Social circumstance report. www.gov.uk/search/all?keywords=mental+health+act+forms&page=4

Gupta, S., Akyuz, E., Baldwin, T., and Curtis, D. (2018, June) Community treatment orders in England: review of usage from national data. *BJPsych Bull.* 42(3): 119–122. https://doi.org/10.1192/bjb.2017.33

Joint Committee (2022) Draft Mental Health Bill. Gov.UK

Mental Health Act (1983) (amended 2007). Online: Mental Health Act 1983.

MHT Practice direction. www.judiciary.uk/wpcontent/uploads/JCO/Documents/Practice+Directions/Tribunals/statements-in-mental-health-cases-hesc-28102013.pdf

Naik, J (2017) A Guide to writing your first mental health tribunal report. www.communitycare.co.uk/2017/03/29/guide-writing-first-mental-health-tribunal-report/

NHS Digital (2022) Mental Health Act Statistics, Annual Figures, 2021-2022 Online: https://digital.nhs.uk/data-and-information/publications/statistical/mental-health-act-statistics-annual-figures/2021-22-annual-figures/community-treatment-orders

NMC (2024) Nursing and Midwifery Council. www.nmc.org.uk/standards/code/

Practice Direction (2013) www.judiciary.uk/wpcontent/uploads/JCO/Documents/Practice+Directions/Tribunals/statements-in-mental-health-cases-hesc-28102013.pdf

Priebe, S. (2021) Patients in mental healthcare should be referred to as patients and not service users. *BJPsych Bull.* 45(6): 327–328. https://doi.org/10.1192/bjb.2021.40

Sullivan, J. (2013) Practice direction, First Tier Tribunal Health Education and Social Care Chamber statements and reports in mental health cases. Tribunals, Courts, and Enforcement Act (2007). www.judiciary.uk/wp-content/uploads/JCO/Documents/Practice+Directions/Tribunals/statements-in-mental-health-cases-hesc-28102013.pdf

SWE (2019) Social Work England. www.socialworkengland.org.uk/standards/professional-standards/

The Mental Health Bill (2025) *Forthcoming.*

Wessely, S., Lloyd-Evans, B., and Johnson, S. (2019) Reviewing the Mental Health Act: delivering evidence-informed policy. *Lancet Psych.* 6(2): 90–91.

13 The Patient, Nearest Relative, and Advocate's Evidence

Amy Rushen

(Please note that for the purposes of this chapter, references to a patient includes patients detained on an unrestricted inpatient basis and patients who are being treated in the community under a Community Treatment Order. This chapter does not reflect law or procedure specific to restricted patients. Any use of "Tribunal Procedure Rules 2008" refers to the Tribunal Procedure (First-tier Tribunal) (Health Education and Social Care Chamber) Rules 2008.)

Introduction

It is important to note from the outset that a patient has two opportunities to put their views to the Tribunal, namely through a Pre-Hearing Examination and through oral evidence, although the patient may choose not to participate in either process.

Pre-Hearing Examinations

A Pre-Hearing Examination (PHE) is an opportunity for the patient to meet with the Tribunal's Medical Member and under r.35(1) Tribunal Procedure Rules 2008, the purpose of a PHE is to allow the Medical Member to form an opinion of the patient's mental condition. Under r.34(2) Tribunal Procedure Rules 2008, PHEs are directed automatically where a patient is detained under s. 2 of the MHA (1983), but require an application to be made on behalf of any other patient. As such, every patient can be afforded an opportunity to meet with the Medical Member outside of the Tribunal hearing itself.

Where a PHE is directed, the Medical Member will make arrangements to meet with the patient before the hearing, either in person or by appropriate video link. The Responsible Authority will have been directed to disclose the patient's progress notes to the Medical Member before that meeting, although in practice, there are occasions where progress notes are not made available. The patient may be accompanied for a PHE, for example, by a member of inpatient nursing staff or the patient's legal representative, but it is permissible under r.34(1) Tribunal Procedure Rules 2008 for that meeting to take place in private if the patient prefers. However, the patient's preference for a private meeting would be subject to the usual risk assessments and would only take place in private if it is safe to do so.

A patient can refuse to participate in a PHE, even where an application has been made by the patient's legal representative. It is the patient's choice whether to attend such a meeting. Where a PHE has been requested and has not taken place for reasons beyond the patient's control, for example, in the case of physical ill health, the patient's representative may seek an adjournment of the hearing so that a PHE can take place. A PHE is particularly important where a patient does

DOI: 10.4324/9781003635543-16

not wish to attend the Tribunal hearing, as it is the only opportunity for the patient to be heard in person by a Tribunal Panel member.

If the patient chooses to attend the PHE, the Medical Member will take the patient through a series of questions focussed on issues relevant to the statutory criteria but will not specifically reference the criteria. The Medical Member will note the patient's responses but will also assess the patient's presentation and mental state.

As part of the Tribunal Panel's discussions before the hearing, details of this meeting will be shared by the Medical Member with other Panel Members. The Panel will take the information into account as part of the totality of the evidence but any view formed or expressed by the Medical Member must be a preliminary view only (*R (on the application of S) v Mental Health Review Tribunal* [2002] EWHC (Admin) 2522). The Medical Member will also give a summary of any progress notes received, usually focussing on notes that cover the period between the date of any reports and the date of the Tribunal hearing.

It is important to note that if a PHE is directed by the Tribunal, it is considered an essential part of the proceedings and patients must be supported when engaging with the PHE. The support offered should be similar to the way in which the patient will be supported in engaging with the Tribunal hearing itself. All parties involved in the Tribunal process are required to help the Tribunal further the overriding objective of dealing with cases fairly and justly (r.2(1) and r.2(4)(a) Tribunal Procedure Rules 2008), part of which is ensuring the patient can, so far as practicable, participate fully in the proceedings (r.2(2)(c) Tribunal Procedure Rules 2008). On a practical note, patients may find it helpful to speak with a Panel Member in a less pressured environment, and may feel more comfortable having met a Panel Member before the hearing itself. It will also assist the Tribunal in focussing its attention on the relevant issues and dealing with the hearing in a way that is proportionate to the issues (r.2(2)(a) Tribunal Procedure Rules 2008).

When the hearing commences, a summary of the PHE will be given to all parties. This summary will include the patient's views, any preliminary view formed by the Medical Member in respect of the patient's mental state, and any matters of note from the patient's progress notes. The PHE summary is usually given at the outset of the hearing before any other evidence is heard, and is generally given by the Tribunal Judge, although on occasion, the PHE summary may be given by the Medical Member. This summary will be given even where the patient has chosen not to attend the Tribunal hearing, or is unable to do so.

The Patient's Evidence

Before a Tribunal hearing, the patient must have sight of any reports filed with the Tribunal. When a patient is represented, the reports will be sent to the patient's representative, who will then share those reports with the patient. However, where a patient is not represented, the reports must be given to the patient directly in good time before the Tribunal hearing. Failure to provide an unrepresented patient with the reports before a hearing may result in a Tribunal hearing being adjourned; the reports are Responsible Authority's written evidence in support of detention and it would be patently unfair to proceed when the patient has not had sight of the case being made by the Responsible Authority.

A patient can choose whether or not to attend a Tribunal hearing; this choice applies irrespective of whether it is an application by the patient or an automatic reference. Where a patient does not attend, the Tribunal can still proceed under r.39 Tribunal Procedure Rules 2008 in the patient's absence. However, in order to do so, the Tribunal must be satisfied that the patient has been notified of the hearing (or that reasonable steps have been taken to notify the patient), and that the patient has decided not to attend or is unable to attend due to ill health (r.39(2)(a)

Tribunal Procedure Rules 2008). Where a PHE has been directed, it must have either taken place or have been deemed impracticable, for example, where a patient has gone AWOL or is too ill to participate safely (r.39(2)(b) Tribunal Procedure Rules 2008). In circumstances where a PHE is not directed, the Tribunal can conclude that it was unnecessary under r.39(2)(b)(ii) Tribunal Procedure Rules 2008. However, even when all the practical requirements have been satisfied, the Tribunal must also satisfy itself that it is in the interests of justice to proceed with the hearing without the patient being present (r. 39(1)(b) Tribunal Procedure Rules 2008).

Where the patient does not attend, the Tribunal will first make enquiries of the patient's legal representative, both in respect of the practical requirements but also in respect of the representative's views on proceeding in the absence of the patient. The patient may have chosen not to attend because there has been an opportunity to speak with the Medical Member in the PHE, or the patient may simply not want to participate. It is incumbent on the legal representative to put forward a view, and the legal representative may seek an adjournment if there have been practical difficulties in securing the patient's attendance, for example, if the patient has been hospitalised for physical health issues.

The Tribunal may also ask for information from inpatient nursing staff or community team members, for example, where there may have been conversations with the patient about attending the hearing. Such conversations are not simply to inform the Tribunal of the practicalities, they should instead be underpinned by the duty to assist the Tribunal in furthering the overriding objective and promoting the patient's participation in proceedings, insofar as is practicable (r.2(1) and r.2(2)(c) Tribunal Procedure Rules 2008).

If a patient does attend, the patient can choose whether or not to give evidence. A patient may choose to present for the hearing but not offer any views or answer any questions. A patient also has the right to give evidence even where the patient may lack capacity to instruct a legal representative, or to consent to a care or treatment plan.

Prior to the hearing, professionals will have filed written evidence with the Tribunal, and copies of that evidence will have been provided to both the patient and any legal representative. The templates provided for the purposes of written evidence will ask for views on any adjustments that are necessary to promote a patient's participation in the proceedings. Professionals should consider the patient's ability (or otherwise) to give evidence when answering this question. This should include consideration of the pressure that the patient may feel when appearing in front of the Tribunal, which may have an adverse effect on the patient's usual presentation. In dealing with cases fairly and justly, the Tribunal must avoid unnecessary formality and seek to be flexible (r.2(2)(b) Tribunal Procedure Rules 2008). Requests for adjustments can be general or can be specific to the patient's current presentation. They may include, for example, adjustment to language used by the Tribunal to ensure that questions are clear and short, a request that the patient be permitted to speak first and leave thereafter, or to make the Tribunal Panel aware that the patient may struggle to listen to the evidence of others. Tribunal Panels will, so far as is practicable, take appropriate steps to promote the patient's participation in proceedings (r.2(2)(c) Tribunal Procedure Rules 2008). Where a patient may require information in easy read format, professionals are encouraged to highlight this need in their reports; the Tribunal written decision and reasons following a hearing can also be produced in easy read format if necessary and appropriate.

Professionals may also be asked to consider a risk assessment prior to a Tribunal hearing; again, any such assessment should consider not just the patient's usual presentation but also how that patient may react to giving evidence and hearing the evidence of others.

The order of evidence in a Tribunal hearing is a matter for the Tribunal Panel to decide, but the Panel will normally seek the views of the patient's legal representative before deciding the order of evidence. A patient will often be heard first, for a number of reasons. It may be the patient's application, hence it being appropriate that the patient's speaks before other parties, but even on a reference, the Tribunal Panel is considering the restrictions on that patient's liberty so may want to hear from the patient first. A patient who is more unwell may struggle to remain in a hearing and if giving evidence last, may feel unable to stay in the Tribunal hearing for that length of time. Patients may also prefer not to listen to the evidence of others and want to speak first so that the patient can then leave. Where a patient has given evidence before professionals, it is usual that the patient is given a right of reply before conclusion of the hearing. However, if a patient expresses a strong wish to be heard at conclusion of the professional evidence, the Tribunal may respect that preference.

Before the patient is heard, a summary of any PHE will be given by the Tribunal Panel and the patient's representative will set out the patient's position, in particular, which areas of the statutory criteria (if any) are being disputed. The patient's representative will then take the patient through a number of questions to elicit the patient's evidence on the areas in dispute. This will include giving the patient an opportunity to correct anything that the patient considers was incorrectly reflected in the PHE summary. Where a patient is unrepresented, the Tribunal Panel will take the role of questioning the patient. The patient's evidence will generally focus on issues relating to the statutory criteria, for example, whether the patient accepts the presence of mental disorder, whether the patient is now well enough to leave hospital or to be discharged from a Community Treatment Order, as well as issues in respect of risk. Where a PHE has taken place, the patient's oral evidence is likely to be more brief, as the patient's views on a number of issues will have already been elicited.

The importance of legal representation for a patient cannot be underestimated; whilst a patient can appoint someone who is not legally qualified to act as a representative, a lay representative may lack the knowledge and understanding to challenge the Responsible Authority's case for detention.

Whilst giving evidence, the patient may occasionally try to engage directly with professional witnesses, or try to involve professionals in answers. For example, a patient may ask the Responsible Clinician to confirm details of medication, or ask the Care Coordinator to explain home circumstances or condition. The Tribunal Panel will redirect the patient in those circumstances and ask that answers are addressed to the Tribunal Panel only; the legal representative will likely also confirm that the relevant information will be elicited from the professional in due course.

If the patient's evidence is heard first then it is likely that the Tribunal will offer the patient the choice whether or not to remain in the hearing for the professional evidence. Should the patient leave, it would be usual for the patient to return after the Tribunal Panel deliberations for announcement of the decision.

It may be difficult for the patient to hear the evidence of others and there are times when a patient may become disruptive. The Tribunal does have the right under r.38(4) Tribunal Procedure Rules 2008 to exclude any person from the hearing where that person's conduct is disrupting, or likely to disrupt, the hearing. Exclusion of a patient by a Tribunal Panel is not a step that is taken lightly, as any exclusion must be balanced against the need to promote the patient's participation in the proceedings (r.2(2)(c) Tribunal Procedure Rules 2008) as well as the patient's broader right to a fair hearing (Human Rights Act 1998, Schedule 1, Part 1, Article 6). In circumstances where a patient has been excluded, the Tribunal Panel may not permit the patient to return to hear announcement of the decision, although clearly, the Tribunal Panel will make arrangements with either the patient's representative or clinical team to convey the decision to the patient.

On occasion, the patient may give evidence in the absence of professionals. This will generally be as a result of an application made by the patient's representative at the outset of the Tribunal hearing; the application is usually because the patient feels unwilling or unable to speak freely in front of professionals. With a younger patient, it may be less intimidating for the patient to speak in front of the Tribunal Panel and representative only. The Tribunal Panel can make a direction to that effect under r.38(4)(b) Tribunal Procedure Rules 2008 if the Panel are satisfied that the presence of professionals may prevent the patient from giving evidence freely. In such circumstances, professionals will be asked to rejoin the Tribunal hearing after the patient has spoken and, if the Tribunal Panel considers it appropriate, a brief summary of the patient's evidence will be provided.

The Nearest Relative

The nearest relative has particular legal status for the purposes of both the Mental Health Act 1983 and the Mental Health Tribunal, and must be consulted as part of the Tribunal process, even when the patient has asked that information is not shared with that person.

The nearest relative is not the patient's next of kin. A patient can nominate anyone to take the role of next of kin, including someone without any legal or blood relationship. However, a nearest relative is defined in s.26 Mental Health Act 1983 and means the first adult from the following list:

(a) Husband, wife, or civil partner;
(b) Son or daughter;
(c) Father or mother;
(d) Brother or sister;
(e) Grandparent;
(f) Grandchild;
(g) Uncle or aunt; or
(h) Nephew or niece.

Where a group is identified, and there is more than one person in that group, the oldest of the group shall be considered the nearest relative. For example, where a patient is unmarried, with no adult children, and living parents, that patient's nearest relative will be the older of the patient's parents. A person will not be considered the nearest relative if that person does not live in the UK (s.26(5) Mental Health Act 1983) and in certain circumstances, including no preexisting marriage between the patient and another person, as well as cohabitation of over six months, an unmarried partner may be treated as a husband, wife, or civil partner (s.26(6) Mental Health Act 1983). There are further complexities to identify a nearest relative in accordance with statute, so advice should be sought from an Approved Mental Health Practitioner (AMHP) where necessary.

Correct identification of the nearest relative is essential for any patient subject to restrictions under the Mental Health Act 1983. A nearest relative has rights defined by statute, including the right to request a Mental Health Act assessment (s.4 Mental Health Act 1983), to apply directly to a hospital for a person to be admitted under section (ss.2 & 3 Mental Health Act 1983), to request that a Responsible Clinician discharge a patient (ss. 23 & 25 Mental Health Act 1983), and to apply to the Tribunal for discharge (s.66 Mental Health Act 1983). The role of the nearest relative therefore acts as a crucial safeguard to the rights of any person subject to the Mental Health Act 1983 and should never be dismissed as "just the next of kin".

Where there is no nearest relative identified (or any nearest relative is unwilling to take on the role), another person can be appointed by the County Court to take on the role. This person is normally a professional, similar to a professional trustee or attorney for those without Mental

Capacity. Occasionally, a nearest relative will have been displaced by the County Court on the basis that the nearest relative was acting without due regard to the welfare of the patient or the public; in these circumstances, someone else will have been appointed to take that role. Where a nearest relative is identified but incapable of acting, for example, through illness or lack of capacity, an application for displacement should be made to the County Court. Applications for displacement are complex but necessary and again, it is usually appropriate to seek advice from an AMHP if circumstances suggest that displacement is necessary.

More commonly, families may have informally delegated the role amongst themselves, for example, a parent who is getting older or who does not have English as a first language will ask a patient's adult sibling to take on the role. Often in these circumstances, families do not understand the importance of the role of nearest relative. Professionals should ensure that families understand the rights and responsibilities of a nearest relative and if a family have agreed that someone other than the nearest relative take on the role, formal delegation should take place. In accordance with Regulation 24 of the Mental Health (Hospital, Guardianship and Treatment) (England) Regulations 2008, this must follow a particular process. The nearest relative must complete a written notification which states that the functions of nearest relative are being delegated to another person and giving that person's details. Such notification must be sent to the patient and either the hospital in which the patient is detained, or in the case of a community patient, to the patient's responsible hospital.

In simple terms, every patient should have a nearest relative who is willing and able to take on the role and exercise the rights of a nearest relative in circumstances where it is in the interests of the patient's welfare to do so.

For the purposes of the Tribunal, the views of the nearest relative will be communicated in one of two ways, either by the patient and professionals passing on those views or by the nearest relative attending the Tribunal hearing in person.

Views of the Nearest Relative

The identity of the nearest relative must be provided to the Tribunal in the Statement of Information prepared by the Mental Health Act Administrator. This ensures that there is early identification of the nearest relative; the Practice Direction: First-tier Tribunal Health Education and Social Care Chamber: Statements and Reports in Mental Health Cases ("the Practice Direction") also requires the Mental Health Act Administrator to confirm if the patient has asked that information is not passed on to their nearest relative, and whether the patient has Mental Capacity to make such a request. It is important to note that whilst a nearest relative has particular rights and responsibilities, these do not override the patient's right to confidentiality. Where a patient has said that no information should be given to the nearest relative, particularly where there has been a breakdown of any relationship, professionals should consider whether delegation or displacement is in the best interests of the patient. However, even where the patient's confidentiality must be respected, the nearest relative can (and must) be consulted.

Given that a nearest relative may be involved in a patient's care and treatment plan, there will likely have been discussions between the nearest relative and the patient's treating team. In accordance with r.15(2)(a) Tribunal Procedure Rules 2008, the Tribunal may admit evidence whether or not the evidence would be admissible in a civil trial in England and Wales. There is therefore no prohibition on hearsay in the Tribunal, although in accordance with *DJ, R (on the application of) v Mental Health Review Tribunal* [2005] EWHC 587 (Admin), the Tribunal must exercise their judgment as to the weight attached to hearsay evidence. Hence, it is permissible for the treating team to relay the views of the nearest relative if asked to do so. The patient may also put forward views from the nearest relative; this is most common where the patient was living with the nearest relative before admission or is seeking to live with the nearest relative when discharged.

Additionally, the Practice Direction specifically requires that the social circumstances report must include the views of the nearest relative. It states that the only exception is where, having consulted the patient, it would be inappropriate or impractical to do so. A prohibition by the patient on information sharing does not automatically render consultation with the nearest relative inappropriate. The views of a nearest relative can be taken without sharing information about the patient, in the same way that professionals will gather information from anyone involved in the patient's care or those who can offer collateral information.

Importantly, where the author of the social circumstances report takes the view that it is inappropriate or impractical to seek the views of the nearest relative, the Practice Direction requires that reasons are given and that the author describes any attempts to rectify matters.

This responsibility is specific to the author of the social circumstances report and is a positive requirement; the responsibility cannot be adequately discharged by simply repeating information garnered from other sources, such as clinical records or an AMHP report. The nearest relative can often offer key information that will be pertinent to the Tribunal, such as information about circumstances of admission, details of any risk incidents, views on whether the patient has reached a baseline following treatment, or their view on the likelihood of the patient remaining concordant with medication and cooperating with professionals if discharged. It should be made clear to the nearest relative that their views will be shared with the Tribunal and the patient. Occasionally, a nearest relative will share views on the basis that such views are not disclosed to the patient. Whilst it is possible under the Tribunal Procedure Rules 2008, in particular r.14(2), to seek an order for non disclosure, the legal test for such an order sets the bar very high. An order for non disclosure may only be made where disclosure be likely to cause serious harm and, having regard to the interests of justice, such an order is proportionate. As such, concerns from a nearest relative that the patient may become upset at hearing any views is highly unlikely to meet the test for non disclosure.

The Nearest Relative at the Tribunal

A nearest relative does have the right to apply to the Tribunal in certain circumstances, including where the nearest relative has requested discharge but it has been blocked by the Responsible Clinician, or where the patient is detained under s.3 or subject to a Community Treatment Order (s.66 Mental Health Act 1983).

Such applications are relatively rare but where an application is made, the nearest relative would have the right to legal representation and would be heard by the Tribunal in the same way as the patient. The nearest relative would also be served with the relevant reports and other documents.

It is far more common that a nearest relative appears in front of the Tribunal as a result of an application or reference in respect of a patient.

In those circumstances, the patient's nearest relative will be sent notice of any Tribunal hearing and will be asked to respond to Tribunal service in respect of attendance. If a nearest relative wants to attend, details of the hearing will be provided, including the link if the hearing is taking place online. It may be possible for the nearest relative to join online with the patient, either on the ward or from whatever venue the patient uses to join an online hearing; otherwise, the nearest relative will join separately. If a nearest relative requires an interpreter, this is not normally arranged by the Tribunal service.

Whilst the relevant reports will be sent to the patient and the patient's representative, they will not be sent to the nearest relative. The reports can only be disclosed to the nearest relative with the consent of the patient.

Attendance of the nearest relative at the hearing is not automatic; a nearest relative is subject to the same powers of exclusion as any other person (r.38(4) Tribunal Procedure Rules 2008). A patient may not want the nearest relative to attend, particularly if the views of the nearest relative do not accord with the views of the patient. In those circumstances, the Tribunal will seek to be flexible (r.2(2)(b) Tribunal Procedure Rules 2008). It may be that the Tribunal directs that the nearest relative attends but does not address the Tribunal, or that the nearest relative addresses the Tribunal without the patient being present. Often, the Tribunal Panel will rely on the patient's legal representative or the professionals to assist with suggestions about how to balance the patient's right to participate against the nearest relative's wish to participate. However, in circumstances where the nearest relative addresses the Tribunal Panel in the absence of the patient, it should be made clear that the views of the nearest relative will be recorded in the Tribunal decision and that decision will be provided to the patient.

Where a nearest relative attends and wishes to address the Tribunal, this will usually take place at conclusion of the other evidence. The patient's legal representative may want to address specific issues with the nearest relative, such as whether the patient will be living with the nearest relative after discharge, or if the nearest relative has a view on whether the patient has returned to baseline, or how support from the nearest relative may mitigate risk. The Tribunal Panel may also want to ask questions of the nearest relative as part of their inquisitorial role. However, in doing so, the Tribunal Panel will bear in mind the fact that the nearest relative is not legally represented and will balance the need to seek necessary evidence against maintaining the relationship between the nearest relative and the patient.

A nearest relative may choose to attend but not speak; it may be that the nearest relative's views are contrary to that of the patient and the nearest relative would prefer not to express those views in front of the patient. There is no legal obligation on the nearest relative to speak to the Tribunal even if present at the hearing and the Tribunal will not force them to do so.

Advocates

Advocates for patients take many forms. Most commonly, a patient will have a legal representative, either chosen by the patient or appointed on the patient's behalf. The role of the legal representative is covered elsewhere and will not be considered below. However, a patient may choose other advocates, including being represented someone who is not legally trained, or to have someone present as an advocate in support, such as a friend, an Independent Mental Health Advocate (IMHA) or an Independent Mental Capacity Advocate (IMCA).

Non-legal Representatives

Unlike the civil and criminal courts, the Tribunal does not require a patient's representative to be a legal representative. As such, under r.11 Tribunal Procedure Rules 2008, a patient can be represented by a lay advocate, although it is an unusual arrangement, particularly given the availability of non-means tested legal aid for persons subject to restrictions of liberty under the Mental Health Act 1983. Lay advocates can be a friend or family member, the nearest relative or a professional such as an IMHA.

Where a patient seeks to be represented by someone who is not a legal representative, the name and address of that representative should be sent to the Tribunal ahead of the hearing.

If this step is taken, then under r.11(3) Tribunal Procedure Rules 2008, the lay representative has the same rights and responsibilities as a legal representative, except for the right to sign a witness statement or application on behalf of the patient. There is also a duty on the Tribunal under r.11(4) Tribunal Procedure Rules 2008 to provide the lay representative with all reports and documents that would be sent to a legal representative.

Where a patient attends a hearing with a representative, and the lay representative's name and address have not been provided in advance, a lay representative can only act for the patient with the permission of the Tribunal.

It should be noted that occasionally, patients will want a fellow patient to act as a representative, oftentimes because there has been discussion about the Tribunal between the patient and the peer. A person who is subject to detention under the Mental Health Act 1983, or who is a community patient, or who is receiving treatment for mental disorder at the same hospital as the patient cannot act as a representative (r.11(8) Tribunal Procedure Rules 2008). However, under r.38(3) Tribunal Procedure Rules 2008, the Tribunal can give permission for the patient's peer to attend in support of the patient, if such attendance does not disrupt proceedings (r.38(4) (a) Tribunal Procedure Rules 2008), or if it promotes the participation of the patient in the proceedings (r.2(2)(c) Tribunal Procedure Rules 2008).

A lay representative will be permitted to ask questions of witnesses in the same way as a legal representative and will be expected to assist the patient in putting forward views to the Tribunal. Lay representatives may be subject to a higher level of intervention from a Tribunal Panel to ensure that the hearing remains focussed on the relevant issues, namely whether the Responsible Authority has made out the statutory criteria in their evidence. A lay representative can also be excluded by the Tribunal under r.38(4)(a) if their conduct disrupts the Tribunal hearing.

Capacity Issues Arising From Appointment of a Lay Representative

The Tribunal Procedure Rules 2008 are clear on the right to be represented by someone who is not a legal representative, subject to compliance with the Tribunal Procedure Rules 2008 and the exclusion of representation by another patient. However, where a patient seeks to be represented by someone who is not a legal representative, the Tribunal may enquire into that decision, to ensure that the decision is a capacitous decision. The patient may be asked to explain to the Tribunal why the lay representative has been chosen, and the reasons for preferring a lay representative rather than a legal representative. A patient may have particular reasons for choosing a lay representative, for example, if a patient has a history of unsuccessful Tribunal applications and has lost trust in legal representatives as a result. A patient's delusions may also prevent the patient from engaging with a legal representative.

Where a Tribunal considers it necessary to review's the patient's capacity to appoint a lay representative then in accordance with s.1(2) Mental Capacity Act 2005, the starting point will be the presumption that the patient has capacity to choose and appoint a lay representative. The Tribunal will want to satisfy itself that the patient understands what a lay representative will be able to do on the patient's behalf, particularly if the lay representative is not a professional such as an IMHA. If the patient has capacity, the Tribunal cannot go against the patient's decision to appoint a lay representative. Where the Tribunal finds that the patient lacks capacity to appoint a lay representative, this does not mean that the patient's lay representative will automatically be displaced in favour of a legal representative. Under r.11(7)(b) Tribunal Procedure Rules 2008, a representative may only be appointed for a patient who lacks capacity if the Tribunal is satisfied that such appointment is in the patient's best interests. In reaching such a decision, the Tribunal would be mindful of the nature of the patient's objections to a legal representative, the distress that imposing a legal representative may cause to a reluctant patient and the effect of such distress on the patient's wellbeing (*YA v Central and NW London NHS Trust and Others* [2015] UKUT 37 (AAC)). As such, the Tribunal may decide that it is not in the patient's best interests to have a legal representative appointed by the Tribunal.

Independent Mental Health Advocates (IMHAs)

Any qualifying patient has the right to the assistance of an IMHA under s.130 A Mental Health Act 1983. For the purposes of that section, a qualifying patient is any patient detained or a community patient (s.130C(2) Mental Health Act 1983). IMHAs are professionals who are specially trained to support patients subject to restrictions under the Mental Health Act 1983, and their role extends far beyond assistance at a Tribunal hearing. The Responsible Authority has a duty to inform patients of their right to an IMHA and subject to the patient's consent, an IMHA has the right to receive information about the patient's care and treatment, as well as being permitted to access the patient's records. The Mental Health Act 1983: Code of Practice ("the Code of Practice") reinforces that the IMHA should play a supportive role in helping patient exercise their rights and participate in decisions that are made about their care (para 6.13 Code of Practice).

There are no provisions that prevent an IMHA from acting as a representative before a Tribunal. However, para 6.14 of the Code of Practice suggests that the role of an IMHA is more appropriately discharged by assisting a patient to seek legal advice and attending any Tribunal hearing in support of the patient, rather than acting as a representative.

Independent Mental Capacity Advocates (IMCAs)

Where a patient has an IMCA, it is likely that the patient also lacks capacity to appoint a legal representative. As such, it would be usual to seek appointment of a legal representative under r.11(7)(b) Tribunal Procedure Rules, subject to the best interests test outlined above. It would be very unusual for an IMCA to act as a lay representative for a patient, as the Chapter 10 of the Mental Capacity Act: Code of Practice emphasises that an IMCA is intended to be a safeguard that sits alongside available legal representation.

Advocates Who Attend in Support of a Patient

More common than a lay representative is an advocate (friend, family, or professional) who attends a hearing in support of a legally represented patient. An advocate, even an IMHA, does not have the right to attend a Tribunal hearing and so the Tribunal Panel will need to grant permission for that person to attend under r.38(3) Tribunal Procedure Rules. It would be very unusual for the Tribunal to refuse the attendance of an IMHA where the patient wants that person to attend, given that an IMHA's professional role is to support the patient's participation.

In those circumstances, advocates will likely be a silent support and play a more active role in supporting the patient during discussions with the patient's legal representative. However, should any advocate, and in particular IMHAs, have any suggestions that would assist the patient in engaging with the Tribunal process, the Tribunal would encourage that the advocate share those views either with the Tribunal directly or with the patient's legal representative.

Conclusion

In considering arrangements for a patient to give evidence, or for the views of the nearest relative to be represented at the Tribunal, there are clearly considerable legal and practical points to consider. However, the underlying purpose of any hearing must also be kept in mind. The Mental Health Tribunal exists for the purposes of reviewing restrictions on a patient's liberty, either by requiring that the patient stay in hospital or by complying with requirements in the community, and which will often include a requirement to take medication, which the patient may not want. For the most part, the patient will be asking for such restrictions to be removed and the role of the Tribunal is to determine whether the restrictions should be removed or not. As such, the patient, as well the patient's nearest relative, have a right to be heard, and must be supported in being heard. From the patient's point of view "justice should not only be done, but should manifestly and undoubtedly be seen to be done" (*R v Sussex Justices, ex parte McCarthy* [1924] 1 KB 256) and the patient's right to participation, support and advocacy is key to achieving the same.

References

DJ, R (on the application of) v Mental Health Review Tribunal [2005] EWHC 587 (Admin).
Mental Health Act 1983.
Mental Capacity Act 2005.
Mental Health (Hospital, Guardianship and Treatment) (England) Regulations 2008.
Mental Health Act 1983: Code of Practice, last updated 31 October 2017.
Mental Capacity Act 2005: Code of Practice, last updated 14 October 2020.
Human Rights Act (1998)
Practice Direction: First-tier Tribunal Health Education and Social Care Chamber: Statements and Reports in Mental Health Cases, 28 October 2013.
R v Sussex Justices, ex parte McCarthy [1924] 1 KB 256.
R (on the application of S) v Mental Health Review Tribunal [2002] EWHC (Admin) 2522.
Tribunal Procedure (First-tier Tribunal) (Health Education and Social Care Chamber) Rules 2008.
YA v Central and NW London NHS Trust and Others [2015] UKUT 37 (AAC).

14 The Legal Representative

Shazad Malik

Introduction

Increasingly people are coming into mental health law from non-legal backgrounds or are in the formative stages of their careers, often building up experience to work in the area of law that they are aiming to eventually specialise in. Due to the enormous impact on the lives of individuals who have not only been deprived of their liberty, but are often receiving powerful medication without their consent in many cases, effective representation is crucial. Paradoxically there is no requirement to be a qualified solicitor or barrister to have rights of audience before the First-tier Tribunal. In order to claim a fee from the Legal Aid Agency legal representatives just need to be a Law Society Accredited Panel Member. The First-tier Tribunal will only appoint Accredited Panel Members to act under Rule 11(7)(a) or Rule 11(7)(b) Tribunal Procedure Rules 2008.

Patient's Rights to Representation

Non-means tested legal aid is available for legal representation before the First-tier Tribunal. This includes nearest relatives who have had their application to discharge the patient barred and wish to exercise their right of application to the First-tier Tribunal. Attendance at Care Programme Approach Meetings and at Hospital Managers Hearings are often rolled into the same file. Means-tested legal aid is available, alternatively clients pay privately, although this is rare. In practise, legal representatives will often assist client's *pro bono* in relation to such meetings, when the means-test requirements are not met.

How Do Patients Decide and Assess Who to Represent Them?

A list of Law Society Accredited Representatives is maintained by the hospital and is provided to patients on the ward. Sometimes relatives or friends contact solicitors on behalf of patients. Patients in longer-stay forensic or rehabilitation settings often rely on recommendations from fellow patients, as they tend to develop closer bonds with them. Some patients determine that they would like to be represented but ask that the tribunal appoints a legal representative on their behalf. In such cases, the tribunal will appoint a Law Society Accredited Panel Member to act under Rule 11(7)(a), (see Appendix A and B). Recent changes to the Legal Aid scheme mean that a Level 1 fee can now be claimed by legal representatives in such cases, even if the patient does not engage and provide instructions. If a capacity statement (MH3) is completed confirming that the patient lacks the capacity to appoint a legal representative, then a Law Society Accredited Panel Member will be appointed under Rule 11(7)(b) to act in the patient's

DOI: 10.4324/9781003635543-17

best legal interests by the tribunal. Legal representatives must remain aware that a client's capacity to instruct can change at any time. What may begin as a Rule 11(7)(a) appointment may change to a Rule 11(7)(b) appointment, and vice versa, (see Appendix A and B).

Once it has been established that a patient lacks the capacity to instruct, the next question is whether it is in the patient's best interest to have representation. It is generally aligned with the overriding objective in Rule 2 of the Tribunal Procedure Rules 2008 to facilitate the patient's participation by asking relevant questions pertinent to the statutory criteria, discussing tribunal reports, and allowing witness questioning.

There are however occasions when it may not be in the patient's best interests. A recent example includes a client who was so distressed by our appointment that a significant portion of a tribunal hearing was devoted to his complaints about our involvement leading to the hearing being adjourned due to lack of time. We subsequently applied for our Rule 11(7)(b) appointment to be rescinded, but our application was refused by a District Tribunal Judge. After additional unsuccessful attempts to engage with our client, we applied again, noting his indication that he was more likely to engage with another firm of solicitors. Thankfully, this was granted.

It is important to keep the situation under review and make another application if further information becomes known. In this case, the client later expressed a preference for a specific firm of solicitors to assist. We contacted them and confirmed their willingness to act if our appointment was rescinded. We were concerned that our continued involvement in the hearing would be ineffective, likely leading to another adjournment and unnecessary costs to the public purse. Depending upon whether you are instructed or have been appointed to act, your role will change. Guidance is contained within the Law Society Practice Note.

Time Constraints and the Machinations of Seeing Patients in Hospital; and in the Community

Section 2 cases require an immediate response and are akin to being a duty solicitor. As well as the strict timescales for lodging an application, this will often be your client's first admission to hospital so they will require timely advice as to the practicalities of being detained and an understanding of how the hospital operates. Although this should have been undertaken as part of the admission process, the stress levels at the time of admission can result in details being forgotten, which will require re-visiting, and can sometimes be lost in a busy ward environment.

Modern technology enables brief initial instructions to be taken with the client's consent via Microsoft Teams (MS). This allows tight deadlines to be met, for example if instructed to lodge a Section 2 tribunal application, which must be done in the first 14 days. Aside from Legal Aid contractual requirements to see 50% of your clients face-to-face, you should aim to see all your clients in person as this assists in building trust. Telephone instructions cannot replace face-to-face contact; clients should only be denied in-person meetings for compelling reasons, such as illness outbreaks or seclusion.

You cannot claim travel to see clients in the community as they are not detained and can attend at your office. There is an exception for those clients who may have disabilities, for which reasonable adjustments need to be made. You need to consider your safety, and your employer has a duty of care in this regard to you as an employee. You should consider meeting community clients at community mental health team offices if they are unwilling to travel to your offices. MS Team meetings may also be an option in cases where clients may have tested positive for a transmissible illness.

Obtaining Instructions

From taking initial instructions to the end of the case, one must be aware of and implement the Legal Aid Agency's Peer Review Guidance. This reflects best practice and is the standard by which firms are assessed and rated.

What Are the Practical Issues Involved?

It is advisable to use an initial client instruction sheet to ensure that key information is obtained as soon as possible. It is important to quickly identify relevant information, i.e. Who is the nearest relative, and do you have permission to contact them? Who is the patient's GP? If the patient was in police custody prior to the admission, consider writing to the custody sergeant for a copy of the custody record if there is a factual dispute as to what occurred in custody.

It is always important to obtain information with the utmost sensitivity. When trying to identify his nearest relative a former client became very defensive and aggressive when his grandmother was mentioned. As a trainee solicitor, I had been left in a room at the end of a long corridor, unsupervised by staff. I had not been provided with a personal infrared transmitter (PIT) alarm. I had to be assertive and stand up when he raised his fists to prevent an assault. Having said that I have only encountered two or three similar incidents over a twenty-year career of representing, and in my experience most patients pose more of a risk to themselves than others.

It is advisable to have a grasp of basic self-defence techniques. "Breakaway training" is offered to nursing staff. To minimise the risks, always speak to staff before seeing your client to identify any risk issues. Sit closer to the door. Ask for a PIT alarm. Make sure there are no objects in the room that could be used to cause injury, such as a mug. Ask staff to remain outside the door if required.

Issues of risk are much more at the fore than in previous years. Following a serious assault on a Judge in another jurisdiction, there was a period where face-to-face hearings were suspended in some hospitals and Trusts. There has been recent judicial guidance relating to face-to-face hearings, which I will mention in the preliminaries section below. There is now a greater reflection in hospitals and wider society as to the concept of safety.

There are occasions when a client may be subject to continuous observations in which case a member of staff may be present during your meetings. It is important to remind staff to keep any discussions confidential and ask them to sign their agreement in writing and not to document your discussion in the medical records. In this situation it is better to be as brief as possible and only obtain basic instructions, with a view to visiting the client again for a more in-depth discussion when the observation levels have been reduced.

Are There Differences in Approach in Representation Between Restricted and Unrestricted Patients?

In each case the focus will be on the statutory criteria. Leaving the legal differences aside, section 2 cases often have more gaps in information as they more often concern patients who are previously unknown to services. Patience is required to advise as to the practical aspects of a hospital admission and to signpost and involve other agencies or lawyers, as required. It is often difficult to determine the merits of section 2 cases. You need to think about what you are not being told as opposed to what you are being told.

Gaining Patients Confidence, Ensuring that Their Voice Comes Across and They Are Heard

In my experience people who are detained, whether in a hospital or prison have a heightened sense of identifying friends and foes. Detention triggers deep emotions linked to our innate survival instincts when living with people who we have not chosen to live with. I have experienced this whilst representing prisoners across the UK. This was apparent when representing patients who were awaiting prison adjudications and were being housed in segregation units. In mental health units one must be mindful that people are often, 'indefinitely detained'. Hospital Orders are given 'without limit of time', which makes it practically impossible for a person to plan their future. This also applies to other detentions under the Act, such as section 3 which can be renewed indefinitely. As this is the reality of your client's predicament, what can be done to alleviate the situation? As far as possible encourage clients to focus on what is achievable and, in their control, rather than outside it. In discussions with staff and during tribunal hearings, carefully manage your client's expectations and clarify what needs to be achieved before discharge to meet various targets. Ask that your client's progress be marked (for example asking a Tribunal to record progress when discharge is not realistic) to help them navigate and manage the inevitable uncertainty.

At the Tribunal – It Is a Court in an Informal Setting – Is There a Difference in Approach?

There is no perfect 'style', nor should one aim to cultivate a particular style. As mental illness knows no bounds, one must adopt a flexible approach. Be sincere. Simplify your language and be yourself. You should be mindful that the proceedings are inquisitorial, which means that the Tribunal will be actively involved in investigating the facts of the case. This contrasts with the competitive processes between both parties in the adversarial system.

Dealing with Preliminaries, How Does This Help?

Recent judicial guidance has been given regarding the management of tribunal hearings. In face-to-face hearings legal representatives and members of the clinical team should speak to the Tribunal to establish if there are any risk issues relating to the patient's attendance at the hearing and how to manage them.

If your client has an eating disorder or other specific need and requires breaks at set times for snacks, then discuss and agree them with the Tribunal at the outset to enable efficient case management. There is of course a legal duty under the Equality Act 2010 to provide reasonable adjustments. It is always important to focus and narrow the issues in the case from the outset. Tribunals are often listed to deal with two cases per day and appreciate focus and relevance. This will also assist your client in managing the hearing, as unnecessarily prolonged hearings can have an impact on their presentation both during and after the hearing.

It is crucial to speak to the Tribunal in the absence of your client if dealing with Rule 14 non-disclosure issues. Often applications will have been made to the Duty Tribunal Judge prior to the hearing for a non-disclosure direction, which is usually granted pending consideration by the Tribunal on the day of the hearing.

Under Rule 14 (2), the Tribunal may give a direction prohibiting the disclosure of a document or information to a person if-

(a) that Tribunal is satisfied that such disclosure would be likely to cause that person or some other person serious harm; and

(b) the Tribunal is satisfied, having regards to the interests of justice, that it is proportionate to give such a direction.

Decision on Non-Disclosure

In *Dorset Healthcare NHS Foundation Trust v MH* [2009] UKUT 4 (AAC), it was confirmed that the '*starting point is that full disclosure of all relevant material should be given*' (para 20).

It is clear from this case that there are two procedures by which information may be withheld from patients. Firstly, and more commonly, it may be argued that the requirements of Rule 14 are met but third-party documents may also be withheld having weighed the patient's Article 6 rights to a fair hearing and the third party's Article 8 rights to privacy.

The information subject to the current application for non-disclosure contains some limited information relating to a third party. Rule 14(2) provides that;

'*The Tribunal may make an order prohibiting the disclosure of a document or information to a person if;*

The Tribunal is satisfied that such disclosure would be likely to cause that person or some other person serious harm <u>and</u>

The Tribunal is satisfied, having regard to the interest of justice, that it is proportionate to give such a direction'

Serious Harm

The tribunal must be persuaded that disclosure would be *likely* to cause the patient or some other person *serious* harm.

Proportionality

The tribunal will also consider the issue of proportionality and ask itself whether the patient would be able to effectively challenge their detention without knowing the information (*RM v St Andrew's Health Care* [2010] UKUT 119 AAC) and that non-disclosure would hamper their ability to participate effectively in the proceedings and that their Article 6 rights to a fair hearing override the third party's Article 8 rights to privacy. The Tribunal will consider if the information is relevant to the statutory criteria for detention and how relevant the third-party information is.

Unless permission is given by the Tribunal for disclosure, this information must not be disclosed. Any discussions regarding disclosure therefore must be undertaken in the absence of your client. There may also be occasions when one wants to avoid causing unnecessary distress by raising certain issues in the presence of the patient, for example making an application to be appointed under Rule 11(7)(b) Tribunal Procedure Rules 2008 on the basis that the patient lacks the capacity to instruct you. This is sometimes unavoidable due to a fluctuating level of capacity, but if you are aware that there may be an issue the hospital should be asked to complete an MH3 Capacity Statement (reproduced earlier), and an application should be made to the Tribunal prior to the hearing for appointment.

Focus and Purpose of Representation at the Tribunal

The Law Society has produced an invaluable practice note titled, "Representation Before Mental Health Tribunals". (A copy has been reproduced in the Twenty-Seventh Edition of Jones 2024, p.996-1015).

In essence, the legal representative has a clear role to act on their client's instructions where the client has capacity to instruct them. The purpose is to advance your client's case (usually for a discharge from detention). One way to do this is to develop a case plan. You can create a grid, or whatever format works for you. The strengths and weaknesses of the case need to be identified, with reference to the statutory criteria. Once they have been established a strategy needs to be formulated to accentuate the strengths and mitigate against the weaknesses.

Professional judgement and skill enable a clear strategy to be pursued by assessing how your client is likely to react during examination-in-chief and in formulating closed questions by way of cross-examination for the professional witnesses. This is why it is important to spend time speaking to your client before the hearing to assess how they are likely to react to proposed questions. If you feel that they are likely to react badly, don't ask the question. Your role is not to conduct a clinical examination or to showcase your advocacy skills.

The opening submission should try to narrow the issues as far as possible and confirm the suggested order of evidence. This is not limited to the statutory criteria alone. If you have obtained independent evidence, you should try to encourage your expert to speak to the professional witness from the Responsible Authority prior to the hearing to try and identify areas of agreement. This can save considerable time and will surely be appreciated by the Tribunal.

The closing submission should have a clear focus on the statutory criteria. You need to outline your client's case and identify hooks to hang it on. Tribunals do not want to hear generic arguments; they need to be tailored to the evidence in the case. If you are asking for discretionary powers to be used, then say why rather than just reminding the tribunal that they have a discretionary power of discharge. For example, if a person is terminally ill and, on an end-of-life care pathway you may wish to advance a case based on discretionary powers. If there are tricky legal arguments to be made, then always prepare and submit a skeleton argument and provide copies of any case-law that you are seeking to rely upon in advance of the hearing. You need to consider and identify the key points from the case-law and apply that to the circumstances of the case. Say why it is applicable and relevant.

The legal representative also has a clear duty to the Tribunal. The Tribunal must not be misled. In accordance with the overriding objective in Rule 2(4)(a) and (b) of the Tribunal Procedure Rules 2008 parties must assist the Tribunal in achieving this objective and cooperate fully.

I like to aim for a "Goldilocks approach" to advocacy. Not too hard and not too soft. There is no need to, "gild the lily". We are dealing with professional witnesses who are acting in the best interests of your client. Advocacy must not become a points scoring exercise. You need to know when to stop. The soft aspect is framing questions, whilst being mindful of the therapeutic relationship. The harder aspects relate to challenging inaccuracies in reports and the sources of information. If it is alleged that your client has been "inappropriate", what does that mean? What is the source of the information? These aspects should be borne in mind when attending Care Programme Approach and Hospital Managers meetings, and in interactions with members of staff.

You must remain mindful that staff are often working in an under resourced system that is still reeling from the aftermath of the pandemic. Healthcare staff often enter their professions committed to helping others, but often find themselves overwhelmed. Be kind to people, whilst advancing your client's case. The individuals you represent have enough challenges without adding unnecessary negative emotions. Adopt a calm and measured approach. Your mind must remain active and sharp, but you must convey a serene demeanour. Don't forget to smile and show your humanity.

The Reports – Making Sense of Incomplete Information

It is important to identify incomplete information and try to obtain it prior to the hearing. You may wish to speak to friends or relatives. Consider obtaining police custody records if there is a dispute or write to the GP to obtain medical records. Approved Mental Health Professional Reports are not always provided as part of the Responsible Authority's case but can often provide useful information or leads to explore further.

If other solicitors are involved, for example in relation to ongoing criminal or family law proceedings, write to them to obtain further information as this could be critical to the outcome of the case. I recently applied to adjourn a section 2 case where there was a fleeting reference to bail conditions preventing the client returning to her home address as well as proposed childcare proceedings to take her children into care. Her application to the Tribunal was to be discharged to return to her home address and look after her children. She was unaware of any bail conditions. Upon discussing the Tribunal reports, she was able to see that we needed further information for her to have a fair and just hearing and agreed with my application to apply to adjourn.

My application to adjourn was successful, and directions were issued for the allocated social worker to investigate and provide further information on bail conditions and childcare proceedings to the tribunal. We also undertook further investigations in relation to legal advice and representation in relation to pending proceedings.

Expectation and Outcome

Always manage your client's expectations. When considering the merits of the case do not be too eager to give detailed advice without having seen the tribunal reports or medical records. It may be that the merits of the case only become clear once you obtain other evidence. It's important to assess the merits of the application as soon as possible to advise your client regarding the best timing of the application.

Semiotics – Hypervigilance, Communication – Tonality, Reading into the Questions, Looking for Signs of Possible Outcome – Reading Body Language of the Panel

On all the advocacy courses that I have undertaken we have been told to "Know thy Judge". I recall an era where Tribunal Panel members' details were not being provided and this was not seen as important. The current practice is for details to be provided and although all Tribunals will consider the statutory criteria, you should be mindful of who you are appearing before and adjust your style and questions accordingly. You need to hear what is not being said instead of only focusing on what is being said. This ability will develop with time and experience.

Giving False Hope and Raising Expectation

One of my former clients who had been detained under a section 37/41 Hospital Order contacted me after his discharge to persuade me to purchase a book that he had written. I did and was particularly interested to read his musings on my role as his legal representative. Unbeknown to me he had carefully observed my body language to try to gauge whether I thought that he would be conditionally discharged. He concluded that I was non-committal and did not give anything away! I felt a sense of relief that I had not inadvertently given him a false sense of hope, enabling him to accept the decision and challenges in his case, many of which were out of his control.

Post Hearing – The Written Reasons

The written reasons for the decision should be provided within three working days in section 2 cases and within seven clear days in all over cases. There are provisions to extend the time-limits. The reasons should explain the Tribunal's findings in relation to the evidence that was presented. Judges are encouraged to draft adequate and concise decisions. The decision should focus on controversial issues in the case. Each party should understand why it won or lost. All the evidence in the case does not need to be rehearsed. The Tribunal does not have to elaborate at length on points of law or explain every step of its reasoning. Guidance was issued by the Senior President on 4 June 2024, which references the relevant case law principles. Written reasons should be discussed with clients in person or over the telephone. Or not at all. It depends upon the client's preference and their state of mind.

The Debrief – Emotional and Psychological Impact of the Outcome

Always try speaking to your client after receiving the oral decision which will usually be given on the day of the hearing. In cases where there are risk concerns it may be given to you as the representative, in the absence of your client. It is a question of judgement in each case when you should speak to your client. The outcome and key points from the hearing should be confirmed in writing. At this stage, the reasons will often be unclear, so do not try to speculate. Wait until you receive the written reasons and ensure that the client is clear as to the timescales for receipt of the decision. Re-assure clients that you will monitor the timescales and chase up as required.

After a successful discharge, one client said, "You have only done half a job." I was bemused at hearing this and upon enquiring as to why, he told me that he wanted a "cast-iron guarantee" that will never be admitted to hospital again! I explained that was not possible and that I could not guarantee that I would not require a future admission to a mental health hospital. There is no shame in needing help and support and clients must not feel that they have 'failed' in any way. Mental health issues can affect people from all backgrounds. Keeping this firmly in one's mind keeps a person grounded and humble.

The emotional effect on the legal representative is often overlooked. Hospital staff often speak freely to colleagues and work in a collegiate atmosphere where decisions are made as part of a Multi-Disciplinary Team. This is often not the case when acting as legal representative as you will be dealing with the case from initial instructions to tribunal advocacy. As an accredited mental health representative, you will often conduct the case with minimal supervision and input from other members of your team. It is important to ensure that you can speak to somebody in your team about your cases to avoid over-identification and burn-out. Although different terms have been used to articulate what happens during the client and representative encounter, it is important to maintain professionalism and appropriate boundaries at all times and seek support when necessary. I recall reading an interesting article by Stephanie Cobb, Clinical Psychologist who concluded her work by quoting William Shakespeare in Romeo and Juliet, "That which we call a rose, by any other name would smell as sweet".

I once saw a triangle entitled, "The Drama Triangle" that had been drawn on a whiteboard in a ward manager's office. I researched this concept upon returning to my office and learnt to always avoid becoming part of this triangle. I have seen the roles of Persecutor, Rescuer and Victim change within the course of a Tribunal hearing. A nearest relative attended as a Rescuer, but then became highly critical of the patient after hearing her evidence and became the Persecutor. By the end the patient had switched roles from Victim to Persecutor and the nearest relative had become the Victim. I encourage you to research this concept and escape conflict. This gives an insight into why legal representatives often refuse to act for both patients and nearest relatives despite there being no actual conflict. It is often due to the significant potential for a conflict of interests arising.

Many years ago, I successfully argued a discharge after obtaining an independent psychiatric opinion. My client was a junior doctor who had some training in psychiatry. I recall visiting him at his home address whilst he was on section 17 leave and met his mother who was understandably proud of her son. He was the first member of his family to attend university. A few weeks after discharge he died by suicide.

Another client who was not discharged was later granted unescorted section 17 leave. She later died in horrific circumstances. It was a suspected suicide and led to an inquest. I remember staring at her file, filled with grief, after the hospital informed me of her death. Having known her for over a decade since her first admission, the news was deeply affecting. By chance, I spoke to the Responsible Clinician a few days later and found her to be warm and reassuring, offering much-needed support. It was at this point that I discovered the concept of over-involvement and over-identification and it was invaluable to talk about what had happened. It is important to note that the Law Society do offer support services for issues, including mental health, whether it is work-related or non-work related.

Appealing the First-Tier Tribunal's Decision

The forms that you will need to use are Forms P9 and P10 which can be accessed via the Government Website. Please read Rule 44, Rule 45 and Rule 46 of the Tribunal Procedure Rules 2008. In summary, clerical errors can be corrected under the, 'slip rule'. The First-tier Tribunal (FTT) can set aside and remake a decision due to procedural irregularities. The FTT can review cases where there has been an error of law and can remake the decision or remit it for reconsideration. Permission can be sought from the FTT to appeal to the Upper-tier Tribunal (UTT) on a point of law. If permission is refused, then an application can be made to the UTT. There are mechanisms to appeal further by way of Judicial Review and to the Court of Appeal.

I have seen little appetite for appealing to the UTT amongst legal representatives. The reasons are mainly twofold. Firstly, there is no extra fee for drafting the grounds of appeal, which can take several hours. Secondly, if for example a section 2 patient has been regraded to section 3 and therefore has a fresh right of application to the FTT, it is sometimes a more pragmatic approach to simply lodge that application rather than deal with the uncertainty of appealing the original FTT decision. Clients often do not have the appetite to deal with further uncertainties and are sometimes reluctant to instruct legal representatives to appeal against FTT decisions. Given their circumstances, it is easy for them to become despondent. Appeals are often impractical in section 2 cases when a client is towards the end of the detention period. Nevertheless,

I have been involved in two successful appeals in the last 12 months, both based on incorrect identification and justification of 'degree' in section 2 cases. In one case the only finding relating to degree was that the patient was, "guarded", with no concurrent nature argument having been made by the Responsible Authority. You need to be wary of risk concerns influencing the Tribunal's decision and effectively, "putting the cart before the horse." It is cases such as these that sometimes allows intellectual dishonesty to creep into decisions. You must remain vigilant and challenge it.

Conclusion

This area of law is not necessarily well-paid, but it is rich in terms of forming character. You will be using your legal skills to provide a voice for some of the most disadvantaged people in our society. You will have a prominent level of client involvement and will often be dealing with the case from taking initial instructions, to representing before the First-tier Tribunal, and beyond. The issues will be medical and social, as well as legal. You will meet people from all religious and cultural backgrounds and of various age-groups, as mental illness knows no bounds. What you experience will undoubtedly leave a lasting impact. There is never a dull day. You will never be lost for words and will always have a story to tell. The stories that you tell will become a source of strength and inspiration for others.

References

English v Emery Reimbold [2002] EWCA Civ 605 at [16].

Flannery v Halifax Estate Agencies Ltd [2000] 1 WLR 377 (CA).

Jones v Jones [2011] EWCA Civ 41 at [3].

Jones, R. (2024). *Mental Health Act Manual*, 27th edn. www.judiciary.uk/face-to-face-hearings-suspen ded-in-some-mental-health-hospitals-and-trusts

South Bucks v Porter [2004] UKHL 33 at [36].

SSHD v TC [2023] UKUT 164 (IAC) Annex para 8.

www.lawsociety.org.uk/career-advice/individual-accreditations/mental-health-accreditation

www.bps.org.uk/psychologist/what-passes-between-client-and-therapist

www.gov.uk/government/collections/mental-health-tribunal-forms

www.lawgazette.co.uk/news-focus/news-focus-mental-health-lawyers-are-willing-to-strike-over-pay/ 5116036.article

www.lawsociety.org.uk/topics/client-care/conflict-of-interests

www.lawsociety.org.uk/contact-or-visit-us/helplines/other-support-services

www.legislation.gov.uk/uksi/2008/2699

www.lawsociety.org.uk/topics/private-client/representation-before-mental-health-tribunals

www.legislation.gov.uk/uksi/2008/2699

*YA v Central and Northwest London NHS Trust. (2015). https://assets.publishing.service.gov.uk/media/ 603e6d278fa8f577c44d659b/Mental_Health_Guide_Quality_February_2021.pdf

Appendix A

Difference between being instructed and being appointed

The key issue here is capacity to appoint a legal representative. As this is so fundamental and should be kept under constant review, I have reproduced the MH3 Capacity Statement below:

1. Is it more likely than not that the patient understands and can retain for the length of your discussion what a tribunal hearing is?

   YES ☐   NO ☐

- That the patient can choose a legal representative who specialises in mental health tribunals and who will be able to offer free legal representation
- That a specialist solicitor will know the relevant law and be able to argue the patient's case at the tribunal
- That a representative will be able in the tribunal hearing to question and challenge the clinical team and say what the patient's views are
- That the patient may not be able to do so as well because of their personal involvement
- That a possible consequence of not being represented is that the patient may have a lower chance of being discharged

Is it more likely than not that the patient can understand <u>all</u> of the above information, retain it for long enough to make a decision, and weigh this information in the balance when making a decision whether to have a representative?

YES ☐   NO ☐

If your answer is NO, please explain why not in more detail (use a separate sheet if needed)

Reason(s) why not:

2. Can the patient communicate their decision sufficiently clearly to be understood?

YES ☐   NO ☐

If you have answered YES to all of the above questions, the tribunal will follow the legal presumption of capacity and assume that <u>the patient DOES have the mental capacity at this time to make a decision as to whether or not they wish to be represented.</u>

If <u>any</u> question in SECTION ONE has the answer 'NO', then go to SECTION TWO.
If <u>none</u> of the questions in SECTION ONE has the answer 'NO', go to SECTION THREE.
Then, in <u>all cases</u> please complete the DECLARATION at the end.

SECTION TWO:

This section focusses upon the best interests of the patient if you think that they do not have capacity to appoint a legal representative.
   Complete this if ANY question in SECTION ONE has the answer 'NO'. (Please tick the boxes as appropriate and complete with more reasons where asked)

3. If the tribunal finds that the patient does **NOT** have the mental capacity at this time to appoint a representative to act for them before the tribunal, is it your opinion that it <u>would be in the patient's best interests</u> to be represented before the tribunal? (NB: Please see Notes for Guidance below)

YES ☐   NO ☐

If your answer is NO, please give brief reasons. These should include, if the patient has said that they do not want to be represented at the tribunal, their reasons why not (use a separate sheet if needed)

Reason(s):

<u>SECTION THREE</u> – Rule 11(7)(a)

Complete this if NONE of the questions in SECTION ONE has the answer 'NO'
If the tribunal finds that the patient **DOES** have the mental capacity at this time to appoint a representative to act for them before the tribunal, which of the following options best summarises your understanding of

the patient's current wishes. If you don't know whether or not the patient wishes to be represented, it would be helpful if you could find out.

☐   The patient wishes to be represented and has now appointed a representative. If so, please provide details of the representative appointed below.

☐   The patient wishes to be represented and wants the tribunal to appoint someone.

☐   The patient does not wish to be represented.

DECLARATION

I confirm that I am a clinician, nurse or other health or social care professional familiar with the patient and I have had contact with the patient in the past four weeks.

My answers reflect my true opinion as to the likely position.

Name

Date

Your professional role

Date you discussed these issues with the patient

Appendix B

NOTES FOR GUIDANCE

The patient's best interests

The tribunal makes the assumption that it will usually be in the patient's best interests to be represented by a lawyer with appropriate expertise and knowledge of mental health law. The tribunal will only appoint a Law Society accredited legal specialist in Mental Health tribunals who can provide legal aid to the patient.

For example, reasons for why it might be in the patient's best interests include[*]:

a)   The need for a fair and thorough analysis of the reasons for the Section or Order of the Mental Health Act that requires the patient to stay in hospital, or restricts their freedom;

b)   The vulnerability of the patient and what is at stake for that patient;

c)   The need for focus, flexibility and appropriate speed in the proceedings and hearing;

d)   Even with help from the panel members, the patient may not be able to adequately explain their wishes and feelings to the tribunal, or say what they agree and disagree with;

e)   The tribunal itself may face difficulty in dealing with the case fairly and justly if the patient is not represented by a competent lawyer who can question witnesses, challenge the evidence, and make legal submissions that analyse the competing factors in the case.

Exceptionally however, it may not be in the patient's best interests to be represented – if, for example, the patient is likely to be caused serious and profound distress by not having their wishes respected and by having representation forced upon them – or if a representative being appointed against their clear wishes means that the patient will refuse to engage or participate in the tribunal process.

Index

For Product Safety Concerns and Information please contact our EU
representative GPSR@taylorandfrancis.com
Taylor & Francis Verlag GmbH, Kaufingerstraße 24, 80331 München, Germany

www.ingramcontent.com/pod-product-compliance
Lightning Source LLC
Chambersburg PA
CBHW080133270326
41926CB00021B/4466